Table of Contents

INTRODUCTION ....
    Why EMDR Matters: Transforming Trauma Therapy 6
    How to Use This Handbook 8

PART 1: FOUNDATIONS OF EMDR THERAPY 11

CHAPTER 1: THE SCIENCE BEHIND EMDR 12
    1.1: Understanding the Adaptive Information Processing Model 12
    1.2: The Role of Bilateral Stimulation in Trauma Processing 15
    1.3: Key Research Supporting EMDR Therapy 17

CHAPTER 2: THE EIGHT PHASES OF EMDR 19
    2.1: Client History and Treatment Planning 19
    2.2: Preparation Techniques for Client Readiness 21
    2.3: Phase 3 Assessment: Target Memory and Emotions 23
    2.4: Desensitization via Bilateral Stimulation 25
    2.5: Integrating Positive Beliefs 27
    2.6: Body Scan for Tension Resolution 29
    2.7: Closure Techniques for Client Stabilization 31
    2.8: Reevaluation Process in Therapy 33

CHAPTER 3: ESSENTIAL TOOLS FOR EMDR THERAPISTS 36
    3.1: Building Rapport with Clients 36
    3.2: Setting Expectations for EMDR 38
    3.3: Preparing Clients for EMDR Sessions 40

PART 2: TREATING TRAUMA WITH EMDR 43

CHAPTER 4: STANDARD PROTOCOLS FOR PTSD 44
    4.1: Selecting Trauma Targets 44
    4.2: Managing Flashbacks with EMDR 47
    4.3: Single-Event vs. Complex Trauma Approaches 49

CHAPTER 5: DISSOCIATION CHALLENGES AND SOLUTIONS 51
    5.1: Understanding Dissociation in EMDR Therapy 51

    5.2 Grounding Techniques for Stabilization 54

    5.3: Identifying and Addressing Dissociative Subsystems 57

PART 3: ADAPTING EMDR FOR COMPLEX CASES 59

CHAPTER 6: TAILORING EMDR FOR COMPLEX PTSD 60

    6.1: Recognizing Signs of Complex Trauma... 60

    6.2: Adjusting Protocols for Safety and Tolerance 63

CHAPTER 7: NAVIGATING THERAPY BLOCKS 66

    7.1: Identifying and Resolving Cognitive Blocks... 66

    7.2: Strategies for Overcoming Resistance... 69

CHAPTER 8: EMDR AND COMORBID CONDITIONS 72

    8.1: Working with Anxiety Disorders 72

    8.2: Integrating EMDR for Depression and Addictions 75

    8.3: Managing Clients with Somatic Symptoms... 77

PART 4: REAL-WORLD CLINICAL APPLICATIONS 79

CHAPTER 9: CASE STUDIES AND PRACTICAL EXAMPLES 80

    9.1: Single-Event Trauma Treatment in Adults 80

    9.2: Complex PTSD with Dissociation... 83

    9.3: EMDR for First Responders with Chronic PTSD 85

PART 5: THE EMDR THERAPIST'S TOOLKIT 88

CHAPTER 10: SCRIPTS FOR EMDR SESSIONS 89

    10.1: Safe/Calm Place Script... 89

    10.2 Grounding Techniques for Dissociative Clients.. 91

    10.3: Installation and Body Scan Scripts 94

    10.4: Incorporating Technology into EMDR Sessions.. 96

    10.5: Guided Mindfulness Scripts for Trauma... 98

CHAPTER 11: ADVANCED TARGET SELECTION FOR EMDR 100

    11.1: Understanding Target Selection in EMDR.. 100

    11.2: Clustered Target Approach for Complex Trauma 102

    11.3: Addressing Implicit and Non-Verbal Memories... 104

    11.4: Targeting Somatic Experiences in EMDR.. 106

THE EMDR PROTOCOLS HANDBOOK

Step-by-Step Strategies for Treating Trauma, PTSD, Dissociation, and Real-World Clinical Cases

Ethan M. Brooks

© 2024 Ethan M. Brooks. The EMDR Protocols Handbook All rights reserved. This book is intended purely for informational purposes. It is provided 'as is' without warranties of any kind, either express or implied. Unauthorized copying, sharing, or distribution of this book, in whole or in part, is strictly forbidden. All trademarks and brand names mentioned herein are the property of their respective owners. The publisher assumes no responsibility for any damages that may arise from the use or misuse of the information contained within this book.

Introduction

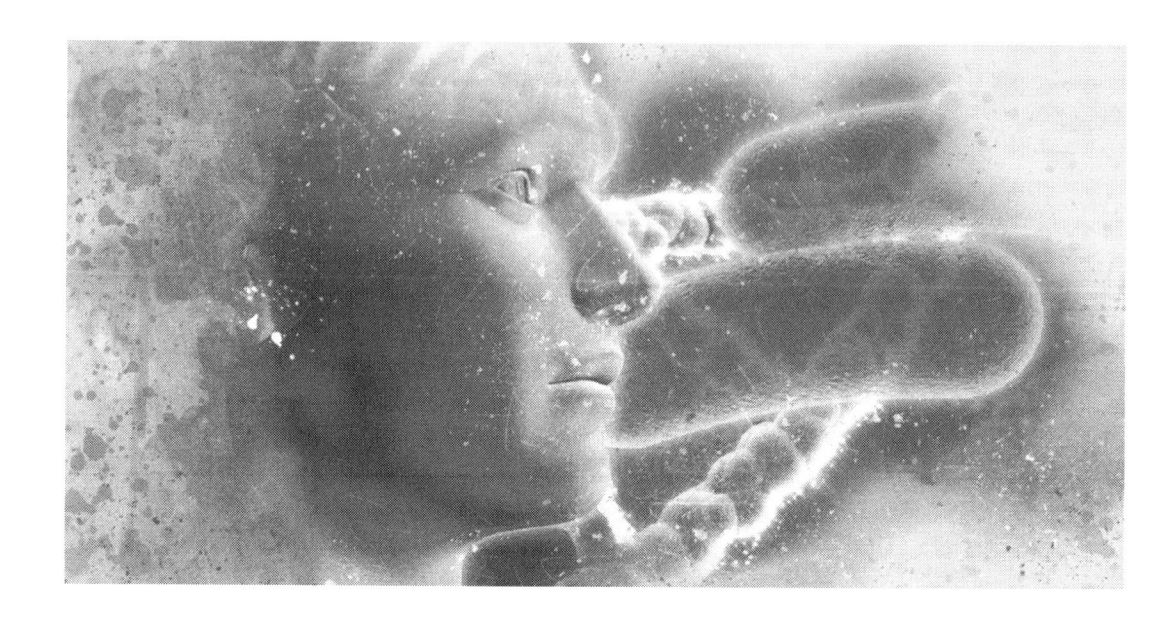

WHY EMDR MATTERS: TRANSFORMING TRAUMA THERAPY

Eye Movement Desensitization and Reprocessing (EMDR) therapy represents a significant advancement in the field of psychology, offering a lifeline to those burdened by the weight of traumatic memories. At its core, EMDR is predicated on the understanding that the mind can heal from psychological trauma much as the body recovers from physical trauma. When you cut your hand, for instance, your body works to close the wound. If a foreign object or repeated injury irritates the wound, it festers and causes pain. However, once the block is removed, healing resumes. EMDR therapy demonstrates that a similar sequence of events occurs with mental processes. The brain's information processing system naturally moves toward mental health. If the system is blocked or imbalanced by the impact of a disturbing event, the emotional wound festers and can cause intense suffering. Once the block is removed, healing resumes. Through EMDR therapy, clinicians help clients activate their natural healing processes.

The efficacy of EMDR in treating post-traumatic stress disorder (PTSD) and other psychological disorders is well-documented, with numerous studies highlighting its ability to reduce the distressing symptoms associated with traumatic memories. Unlike traditional forms of talk therapy, EMDR does not rely on detailed discussions of the disturbing event or extensive exposure to the trauma. Instead, it employs a structured eight-phase approach that includes the use of bilateral stimulation, such as side-to-side eye movements, to help process and integrate traumatic memories into the psyche's adaptive coping mechanisms.

This innovative therapy is particularly transformative for individuals who have found little relief from conventional treatments. For many, EMDR therapy has been a turning point, offering a path out of the darkness of trauma and into the light of emotional healing and resilience. By reprocessing traumatic memories, clients often experience a significant reduction in the power those memories hold over them, leading to a marked decrease in symptoms of anxiety, depression, and PTSD.

EMDR therapy also stands out for its versatility. It has been adapted for a wide range of psychological issues beyond trauma and PTSD, including anxiety disorders, depression, and addiction. This adaptability makes EMDR an invaluable tool in a therapist's arsenal, capable of addressing the complex and varied needs of clients.

The importance of EMDR in transforming trauma therapy cannot be overstated. Its ability to foster rapid and lasting change, often in fewer sessions than traditional therapies, not only benefits clients but also enhances the therapeutic process itself. As therapists, embracing EMDR means equipping ourselves with a powerful method to help our clients navigate the challenges of healing from trauma. It underscores our commitment to providing the most effective, evidence-based treatments available, ensuring that we can meet our clients where they are and guide them toward recovery. Through EMDR, we have the opportunity to witness the profound resilience of the human spirit, as clients reclaim their lives from the grip of trauma and step into a future filled with hope and possibility.

HOW TO USE THIS HANDBOOK

This handbook is meticulously designed to serve as a comprehensive resource for clinicians employing EMDR therapy across a variety of settings and client scenarios. It is structured to progressively build your understanding and application of EMDR, beginning with foundational concepts before advancing to more complex applications and real-world case studies. Each part of the book is crafted to address specific elements of EMDR therapy, ensuring that you have a robust framework to support your therapeutic interventions.

Part 1: Foundations of EMDR Therapy lays the groundwork by introducing the Adaptive Information Processing model and detailing the science behind EMDR, including the role of bilateral stimulation and key research findings. This section is critical for all clinicians, regardless of experience level, as it solidifies the theoretical underpinnings of the practice.

Part 2: Treating Trauma with EMDR delves into the application of standard protocols for addressing PTSD, managing flashbacks, and differentiating between single-event and complex trauma. This section is particularly useful for therapists seeking practical strategies for common trauma-related challenges.

Part 3: Adapting EMDR for Complex Cases explores modifications of the standard protocol to accommodate clients with complex PTSD, navigational blocks in therapy, and comorbid conditions. This part provides advanced strategies for clinicians ready to tackle more challenging clinical scenarios.

Part 4: Real-World Clinical Applications presents a series of case studies and practical examples that illustrate the application of EMDR in diverse contexts. This section is designed to bridge the gap between theory and practice, offering insights into the nuanced application of EMDR strategies.

Part 5: The EMDR Therapist's Toolkit equips you with a collection of scripts, advanced target selection strategies, and guidance on incorporating technology into your sessions. This toolkit is an invaluable resource for enhancing the efficacy of your interventions and navigating complex therapeutic landscapes.

By structuring the book in this manner, we aim to guide you through the intricacies of EMDR therapy, from foundational principles to advanced techniques and practical applications. Whether you are a novice seeking to understand the basics or an experienced practitioner aiming to refine your skills and expand your toolkit, this handbook is designed to meet you at your level of expertise and support your growth as an EMDR clinician.

Part 1:
Foundations of EMDR Therapy

Chapter 1: The Science Behind EMDR

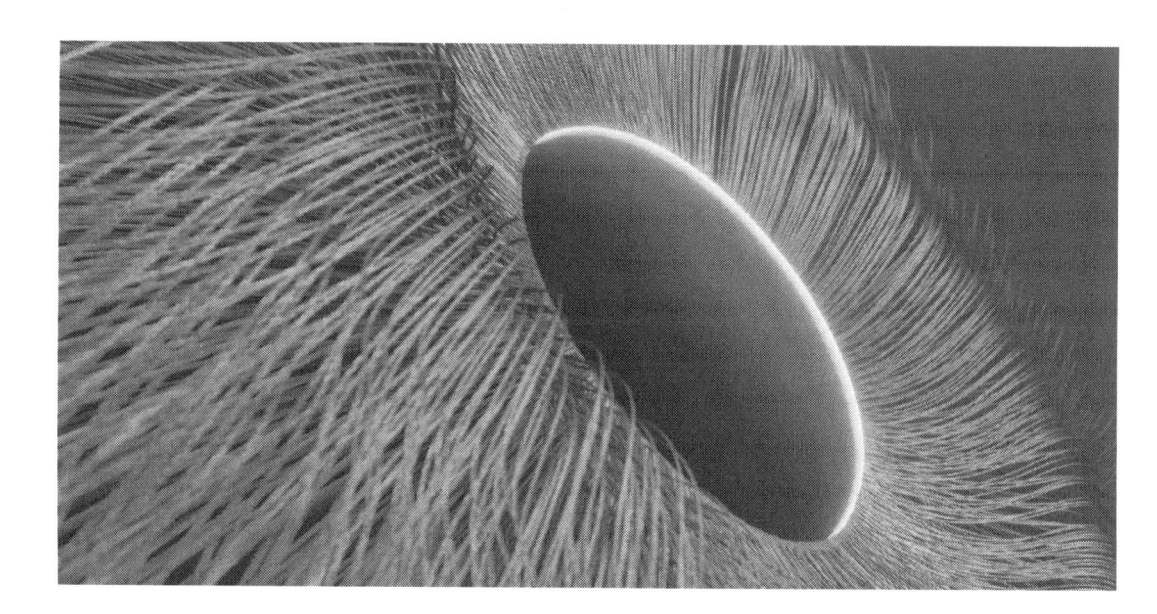

1.1: Understanding the Adaptive Information Processing Model

The Adaptive Information Processing (AIP) model is a cornerstone of Eye Movement Desensitization and Reprocessing (EMDR) therapy, offering a framework for understanding how the brain processes and stores traumatic memories. According to the AIP model, the mind is intrinsically equipped to manage and resolve traumatic experiences. However, when a traumatic event occurs, it can overwhelm the brain's natural processing capabilities, leading to the storage of the memory in an unprocessed, raw form. This unprocessed memory can then trigger emotional and physical responses when similar experiences or reminders occur in the present, often leading to symptoms associated with post-traumatic stress disorder (PTSD) and other trauma-related disorders.

At the heart of the AIP model is the notion that unprocessed memories contain the emotions, thoughts, beliefs, and physical sensations that were present at the time of the traumatic event. These memories are stored in a state that is disconnected from the brain's adaptive learning processes. As a result, they can be easily activated by current situations that resemble or symbolize aspects of the original trauma, leading to distressing symptoms.

Examples of unprocessed memories might include:

- A veteran who hears a car backfire and instantly feels as though they are back on the battlefield, experiencing intense fear and physiological reactions as if the trauma were occurring in the present.

- An individual who was in a car accident and now experiences panic attacks when driving or even when hearing the sound of screeching tires, as these cues activate the unprocessed memory of the accident.

- A person who was bullied in childhood feeling intense anxiety and worthlessness in social situations as an adult, triggered by interactions that echo the dynamics of their childhood experiences.

The goal of EMDR therapy, guided by the AIP model, is to facilitate the processing of these unprocessed memories, allowing them to be integrated into the existing memory network in an adaptive manner. This process involves accessing the unprocessed memory and the associated emotions, thoughts, and physical sensations, and then using bilateral stimulation to help the brain reprocess the memory. As the memory is processed, it is transformed; the distressing emotions are desensitized, negative beliefs are restructured into positive ones, and any physical sensations associated with the memory are resolved. This transformation allows the individual to recall the traumatic event without experiencing the intense emotional and physical responses that were previously triggered by the memory.

The AIP model thus provides a theoretical foundation for EMDR therapy, explaining both the persistence of trauma symptoms and the therapeutic mechanism by which these symptoms can be alleviated. By targeting the unprocessed memories that lie at the root of trauma-related disorders, EMDR therapy can help individuals achieve emotional healing and resolution, freeing them from the grip of their past traumatic experiences.

1.2: The Role of Bilateral Stimulation in Trauma Processing

Bilateral stimulation forms the cornerstone of EMDR therapy, utilizing repetitive left-right stimulation of the brain to facilitate the processing of traumatic memories. This method can include eye movements, auditory tones, or tactile pulses, all designed to engage both hemispheres of the brain. The underlying principle is that bilateral stimulation can mimic the psychological state associated with Rapid Eye Movement (REM) sleep, a phase of sleep during which the brain processes daily emotional experiences. By replicating this natural state of neural functioning during therapy, EMDR facilitates the integration of traumatic memories into the brain's adaptive information processing system.

Mechanisms at Play

The effectiveness of bilateral stimulation lies in its ability to help unclog the emotional processing system of the brain, which can become overwhelmed by trauma. Traumatic events can cause memories to be stored in an isolated, unprocessed form, laden with the original emotional intensity and physical sensations. This can lead to distressing symptoms when the individual is reminded of the trauma. Bilateral stimulation works by activating alternate sides of the brain, helping to stimulate the frozen or blocked information processing system. This process encourages the assimilation and accommodation of the traumatic memories, thus reducing their emotional impact.

Aiding in Trauma Resolution

1. **Desensitization**: Through the rhythmic left-right stimulation, the client's level of emotional distress associated with traumatic memories begins to decrease. This desensitization process is crucial for clients who experience intense emotional reactions when recalling traumatic events. The bilateral stimulation helps to detach the memory from these overwhelming emotions, making the memory less distressing.

2. **Reprocessing**: As the emotional charge of the memory diminishes, cognitive reprocessing becomes possible. Clients are able to reframe and recontextualize the traumatic event, integrating it into their overall life narrative in a more adaptive way. This often involves shifting from a perspective of self-blame or helplessness to one of resilience and empowerment.

3. **Installation**: Bilateral stimulation also aids in the installation phase of EMDR, where positive beliefs are reinforced. For example, replacing a belief such as "I am powerless" with "I am resilient" becomes more effective when the client is in a state of reduced emotional distress and increased neural integration facilitated by bilateral stimulation.

4. **Body Scan**: Following the cognitive and emotional processing of the traumatic memory, clients often proceed to a body scan, where they are asked to notice any residual physical sensations linked to their trauma. Bilateral stimulation continues to play a role here, aiding in the resolution of somatic symptoms associated with the trauma.

Clinical Considerations

When implementing bilateral stimulation, therapists must tailor the approach to each client's needs and responses. Some clients may find certain forms of stimulation more effective or comfortable than others. It is also essential for therapists to monitor the client's level of distress closely, adjusting the pace of therapy accordingly. The goal is to ensure that the client remains within a window of tolerance, where emotional arousal is manageable and does not become overwhelming.

In conclusion, bilateral stimulation is a pivotal component of EMDR therapy, offering a structured, evidence-based approach to trauma processing. By engaging the brain's natural healing capacities, it facilitates the movement of traumatic memories from isolated, distressing experiences to integrated, adaptive narratives. This not only alleviates the symptoms of trauma but also empowers clients, fostering resilience and a sense of mastery over their past experiences.

1.3: KEY RESEARCH SUPPORTING EMDR THERAPY

The empirical support for Eye Movement Desensitization and Reprocessing (EMDR) therapy is robust, with a multitude of studies underscoring its effectiveness in treating post-traumatic stress disorder (PTSD) and complex trauma. Research has consistently shown that EMDR can significantly reduce the symptoms of PTSD, often in a shorter time frame than traditional psychotherapies. This section delves into key studies that highlight the clinical applications and outcomes of EMDR therapy.

Randomized Controlled Trials (RCTs) have been pivotal in establishing EMDR's efficacy. One landmark study compared EMDR to cognitive-behavioral therapy (CBT) in treating PTSD. Results indicated that both therapies produced significant and comparable reductions in PTSD symptoms, but EMDR required fewer treatment sessions. This finding suggests that EMDR is not only effective but also efficient, offering potential cost and time savings for both clients and therapists.

Meta-analyses have further reinforced EMDR's standing in the trauma treatment landscape. A comprehensive meta-analysis examining multiple RCTs found that EMDR significantly reduced trauma symptoms and was as effective as trauma-focused CBT. Importantly, these benefits were maintained at follow-up, indicating the lasting impact of EMDR on reducing PTSD symptoms.

Studies on Complex Trauma have explored EMDR's application beyond single-incident PTSD. Research demonstrates that EMDR is effective in treating complex PTSD, characterized by prolonged exposure to traumatic events and often accompanied by additional symptoms such as emotional dysregulation and dissociation. EMDR's phased approach and ability to process multiple facets of traumatic experiences make it particularly suited for addressing the multifaceted nature of complex trauma.

Neurobiological Research provides insight into the mechanisms underlying EMDR's effectiveness. Functional magnetic resonance imaging (fMRI) studies have shown that EMDR therapy can alter activation patterns in brain regions associated with the processing of traumatic memories, such as the amygdala and hippocampus. These changes are thought to reflect the processing and integration of traumatic memories, supporting the Adaptive Information Processing model central to EMDR.

Clinical Case Studies offer real-world examples of EMDR's transformative potential. For instance, case reports have documented the successful use of EMDR in treating individuals with long-standing PTSD symptoms that had not responded to other treatments. These cases highlight EMDR's ability to facilitate breakthroughs in cases where traditional therapies had been ineffective.

Research on Dissociation underscores the importance of EMDR's preparatory phases in stabilizing clients before trauma processing. Studies have shown that EMDR can be safely and effectively used with clients experiencing dissociative symptoms, provided that appropriate grounding and stabilization techniques are employed. This research emphasizes the adaptability of EMDR to meet the needs of clients with complex clinical presentations.

In summary, the body of research supporting EMDR therapy is substantial and growing. From randomized controlled trials and meta-analyses to neurobiological studies and clinical case reports, the evidence consistently affirms EMDR's efficacy in treating PTSD and complex trauma. As research continues to unfold, EMDR's role in trauma therapy is increasingly recognized, offering hope and healing to those affected by trauma.

Chapter 2: The Eight Phases of EMDR

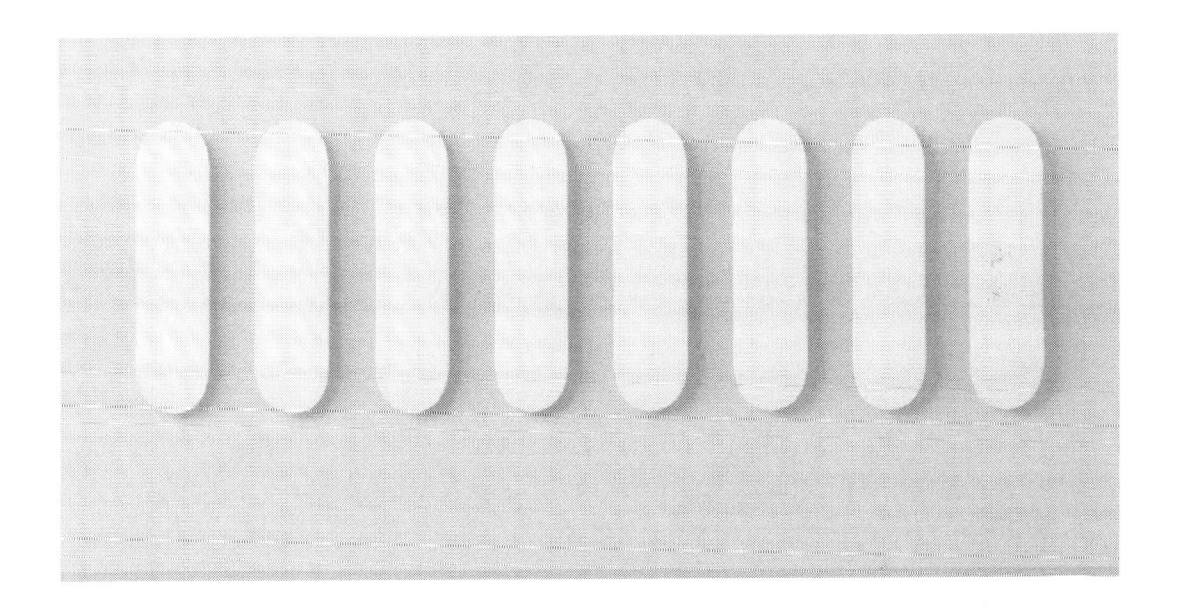

2.1: CLIENT HISTORY AND TREATMENT PLANNING

In the initial phase of Eye Movement Desensitization and Reprocessing (EMDR), gathering a comprehensive trauma history is paramount. This foundational step involves a meticulous process of interviewing the client to uncover the breadth and depth of traumatic experiences that contribute to their current psychological state. It is during this phase that the clinician establishes a rapport with the client, setting the stage for a therapeutic alliance that is crucial for the success of the treatment.

To effectively collect trauma history, therapists should employ a structured yet flexible approach, allowing for the exploration of the client's life narrative. This includes identifying significant life events, both positive and negative, that have shaped the client's psychological landscape. It is essential to approach this task with sensitivity and patience, as recalling traumatic events can be distressing for clients. Therapists must be adept at navigating these conversations with empathy, providing support and reassurance as needed.

Identifying treatment goals is another critical component of this phase. Goals should be collaboratively established, ensuring they are aligned with the client's aspirations for therapy. This involves a clear articulation of what the client hopes to achieve through EMDR, such as reducing the intensity of trauma-related symptoms, enhancing emotional regulation, or improving interpersonal relationships. Setting specific, measurable, achievable, relevant, and time-bound (SMART) goals can facilitate a focused and effective therapeutic process.

Prioritizing targets for EMDR sessions is a strategic process that requires careful consideration. Therapists must discern which traumatic memories to address first, taking into account factors such as the client's current stability, the severity of distress associated with each memory, and the potential for each target to contribute to the client's overall recovery. This prioritization is informed by the Adaptive Information Processing model, which posits that processing these targeted memories can lead to a reduction in trauma-related symptoms and an enhancement of psychological well-being.

In sum, Phase 1 of EMDR therapy lays the groundwork for the subsequent phases of treatment. By thoroughly collecting trauma history, identifying treatment goals, and prioritizing targets, therapists can tailor the EMDR process to meet the unique needs of each client. This meticulous preparation is essential for facilitating trauma processing and fostering recovery, embodying the therapist's commitment to supporting the client through their healing journey.

2.2: PREPARATION TECHNIQUES FOR CLIENT READINESS

Building client readiness is a pivotal aspect of the EMDR therapy process, ensuring that individuals are both psychologically and emotionally prepared to engage in the intensive work of trauma processing. This preparation phase is not merely about informing the client about the mechanics of EMDR but also about equipping them with the necessary tools to manage the emotional upheavals that might arise during the course of therapy. To facilitate this, several techniques and exercises can be employed to enhance client readiness.

Calming Exercises: It is essential to introduce clients to calming exercises early in the therapy process. These exercises serve as valuable resources for clients, enabling them to regain a sense of control and calm when faced with distressing emotions or memories. Techniques such as deep breathing, guided imagery, and progressive muscle relaxation can be particularly effective. For instance, guiding a client through a deep breathing exercise, where they focus on slow, deliberate breaths, can help modulate physiological arousal and induce a state of calm. Similarly, progressive muscle relaxation, which involves tensing and then relaxing different muscle groups, can reduce physical tension and anxiety.

Explaining the EMDR Process: A thorough explanation of the EMDR process is crucial for demystifying the therapy and setting realistic expectations. This involves a detailed discussion of the eight phases of EMDR, emphasizing the role of bilateral stimulation in facilitating the processing of traumatic memories. It is important to explain how EMDR therapy aims to desensitize the client to distressing memories and reprocess them in a way that reduces their emotional impact. Clarifying that some level of emotional discomfort may be experienced during the sessions but that this is part of the healing process can help clients feel more prepared and less apprehensive.

Building Emotional Stability: Before diving into trauma reprocessing, ensuring that the client has a stable emotional foundation is imperative. This can be achieved through the introduction of coping strategies and emotional regulation techniques. Teaching clients skills such as mindfulness, which encourages present-moment awareness without judgment, can be particularly beneficial. These skills not only aid in managing emotional distress during

EMDR sessions but also empower clients to handle stressors in their daily lives more effectively.

Creating a Safe Space: Establishing a sense of safety within the therapeutic environment is essential for client readiness. This includes reassurance about the confidentiality of the therapy process and the collaborative nature of EMDR, where the client has control over the pace of therapy. It may also be helpful to introduce the concept of a 'safe place' – a mental imagery exercise where the client visualizes a place where they feel completely safe and calm. This 'safe place' can then be accessed mentally by the client during or outside therapy sessions whenever they feel overwhelmed.

Addressing Concerns and Misconceptions: It is not uncommon for clients to have concerns or misconceptions about EMDR therapy. Taking the time to address these concerns, providing clear and accurate information, can alleviate fears and build trust in the therapeutic process. Whether it's clarifying that EMDR does not involve hypnosis or discussing the evidence supporting its effectiveness, open and honest communication is key.

Incorporating these techniques into the preparation phase of EMDR therapy not only helps build client readiness but also lays a strong foundation for the therapeutic work ahead. By ensuring clients are well-informed, emotionally stable, and equipped with coping strategies, therapists can facilitate a more effective and empowering EMDR process.

2.3: Phase 3 Assessment: Target Memory and Emotions

In Phase 3, Assessment, the focus shifts to meticulously selecting the target memory that will be the centerpiece of the Eye Movement Desensitization and Reprocessing (EMDR) session. This phase is critical as it sets the stage for the therapeutic work that follows, aiming to alleviate the emotional burden associated with traumatic memories. The process involves three primary steps: identifying the target memory, pinpointing the associated emotions, and evaluating the disturbance level. Each of these steps requires the therapist to engage deeply with the client, fostering an environment of trust and openness.

Identifying the Target Memory: The first step is to collaborate with the client to select a specific memory that is contributing to their current distress. This memory should be one that evokes a strong emotional response and is linked to the symptoms the client is experiencing. It is important for the therapist to guide the client through this process with sensitivity, as recalling traumatic events can be challenging. The selection should be made with consideration of the client's stability and readiness to confront the memory. Using the Adaptive Information Processing model as a framework, the therapist helps the client to understand that processing this memory can lead to significant improvements in their emotional well-being.

Pinpointing Associated Emotions: Once the target memory has been identified, the next step is to explore the emotions connected to it. The client is asked to articulate the feelings that arise when they recall the memory, which may range from fear and sadness to anger and shame. This exploration is not merely about naming the emotions but understanding their depth and the impact they have on the client's life. The therapist's role is to validate the client's feelings and help them recognize that these emotional responses are a natural result of their experiences.

Evaluating the Disturbance Level: The final step in the assessment phase is to determine the level of disturbance the target memory causes. This is typically done using a subjective scale, such as the Subjective Units of Disturbance Scale (SUDS), where the client rates their level of emotional disturbance on a scale from 0 to 10. This quantitative measure provides a baseline for the therapeutic work ahead and helps to monitor progress throughout the EMDR process. It is crucial for the therapist to approach this evaluation with empathy, acknowledging the difficulty in quantifying emotional pain while emphasizing the value of this step in the healing journey.

The assessment phase is a foundational component of EMDR therapy, requiring a delicate balance of technical skill and compassionate client engagement. By carefully selecting the target memory, understanding the emotions it evokes, and evaluating the level of disturbance, therapists can tailor the EMDR process to meet the unique needs of each client. This phase not only prepares the client for the reprocessing work to come but also reinforces the therapeutic alliance, building a shared understanding of the goals and expectations for treatment.

2.4: DESENSITIZATION VIA BILATERAL STIMULATION

In the desensitization phase of EMDR, the primary objective is to lessen the emotional impact of the target memory through bilateral stimulation. This technique involves alternating stimulation of the left and right hemispheres of the brain, which can be achieved through various methods such as side-to-side eye movements, tactile taps, or auditory tones. The process is meticulously designed to engage the client in recalling the distressing memory while simultaneously focusing on an external stimulus, thereby facilitating the processing of traumatic memories in a less distressing way.

Bilateral Stimulation Techniques: The choice of bilateral stimulation technique should be tailored to the client's comfort and responsiveness. For some, visual cues such as moving a finger back and forth across the client's field of vision may be effective, while others may respond better to auditory or tactile stimuli. The therapist's role is to introduce these methods gently and gauge the client's response, adjusting the approach as needed to ensure maximum comfort and efficacy.

Safety and Pacing: A critical aspect of this phase is maintaining a safe pace that the client can handle without becoming overwhelmed. The therapist must closely monitor the client's reactions and adjust the intensity and speed of the bilateral stimulation accordingly. This careful pacing helps prevent retraumatization and ensures that the client remains within their window of tolerance throughout the session.

Measuring Progress: Throughout the desensitization process, therapists employ the Subjective Units of Disturbance Scale (SUDS) to assess the client's level of emotional disturbance in response to the target memory. This scale provides a quantitative measure of progress, allowing the therapist and client to track improvements and identify when the memory no longer elicits significant distress.

Integration of Positive Beliefs: As the emotional charge of the memory decreases, therapists guide clients in integrating positive cognitions or beliefs about themselves that are incompatible with the negative emotions previously associated with the memory. This step is crucial for transforming the memory's meaning and impact on the client's self-perception and emotional well-being.

Therapist's Role: Throughout the desensitization phase, the therapist's role is to provide support, guidance, and reassurance. They must create a safe and trusting environment where the client feels comfortable sharing their experiences and emotions. The therapist's ability to empathize, validate the client's feelings, and maintain a nonjudgmental stance is paramount in facilitating effective processing and desensitization.

Client's Experience: It is important for clients to understand that experiencing a range of emotions during this phase is normal and part of the healing process. They may feel relief, sadness, anger, or even temporary increases in distress, but these emotions are indicative of the brain's efforts to reprocess and resolve the trauma. Therapists should prepare clients for this emotional journey, emphasizing the importance of self-care and the use of coping strategies between sessions.

In essence, the desensitization phase is a cornerstone of EMDR therapy, wherein the bilateral stimulation serves as a powerful tool for diminishing the distress associated with traumatic memories. By carefully navigating this phase, therapists can help clients reprocess trauma in a way that promotes healing and fosters resilience, ultimately leading to a significant reduction in trauma-related symptoms and an enhanced sense of emotional freedom.

2.5: INTEGRATING POSITIVE BELIEFS

The transition to Phase 5, Installation, marks a pivotal moment in the EMDR therapy process. Here, the focus shifts from desensitizing the client to distressing memories to actively reinforcing positive beliefs. This phase is crucial for not only alleviating the pain associated with traumatic memories but also for building a foundation of positive self-perception and resilience in the client. The goal is to ensure that these positive beliefs are fully integrated into the client's memory network, effectively replacing the negative cognitions that were previously attached to the traumatic memory.

To achieve this, the therapist begins by collaborating with the client to identify a positive cognition that is both meaningful and directly counters the negative belief associated with the trauma. For example, if a client's negative belief is "I am powerless," a contrasting positive belief might be "I have the power to control my response." It's imperative that the chosen positive belief resonates deeply with the client, as this will facilitate its integration into the memory network.

Once a positive belief is selected, the therapist employs bilateral stimulation, similar to that used in the Desensitization phase. However, in Installation, the focus is on embedding the positive belief into the client's cognitive framework. The therapist guides the client to hold the positive belief in mind while simultaneously engaging in bilateral stimulation. This process is designed to strengthen the association between the memory and the positive cognition, effectively altering the emotional response to the memory.

Throughout this phase, the therapist continuously monitors the client's level of belief in the positive cognition using the Validity of Cognition (VOC) scale, which typically ranges from 1 (completely false) to 7 (completely true). The aim is to progress to a point where the client rates the positive belief as a 6 or 7, indicating strong acceptance and integration of the positive belief.

It is not uncommon for clients to encounter difficulties in fully embracing the positive belief, especially if the negative cognition has been deeply ingrained over time. In such instances, the therapist may need to revisit earlier phases of

EMDR to further process any lingering emotional distress or negative beliefs before continuing with the Installation phase.

The Installation phase is also an opportunity to reinforce the client's sense of safety and control, which is paramount for individuals who have experienced trauma. The therapist might incorporate techniques such as guided imagery or mindfulness exercises to support the installation of positive beliefs and enhance the client's emotional regulation skills.

As the positive belief becomes more integrated, the client should begin to notice a shift in their emotional response to the memory and a reduction in trauma-related symptoms. This signifies a successful reprocessing of the traumatic memory, where the memory no longer elicits significant distress, and the client is able to view themselves and their experiences through a more positive and empowered lens.

The Installation phase is a testament to the transformative potential of EMDR therapy. By meticulously embedding positive cognitions into the client's memory network, therapists can help clients rewrite the narrative of their traumatic experiences, fostering a sense of empowerment and resilience that extends beyond the therapy session. This phase is not only about changing how clients perceive their past but also about equipping them with the beliefs and tools they need to navigate future challenges with confidence and strength.

2.6: BODY SCAN FOR TENSION RESOLUTION

The body scan phase is a critical component of the Eye Movement Desensitization and Reprocessing (EMDR) therapy, focusing on identifying and resolving physical distress that may remain after processing traumatic memories. This phase allows both the therapist and the client to tune into the body's sensations, which can often hold residual stress and tension related to traumatic experiences. The goal is to ensure that the client achieves a state of physical and emotional relief, marking a significant step towards holistic healing.

Initiating the Body Scan: The therapist guides the client to bring their attention to their physical self, starting from one end of the body, typically the feet, and moving gradually towards the head. This systematic approach ensures that no area is overlooked, as clients are encouraged to notice any sensations, including tightness, heaviness, or discomfort, that arise in different parts of their body.

Identifying Residual Tension: As the client shifts their focus through various regions of the body, they are asked to identify areas where they perceive tension or discomfort. This process is not just about recognizing overt pain but also about subtle sensations that may indicate underlying distress. It's crucial for the therapist to remind the client that there is no right or wrong sensation to experience and that the objective is to observe and acknowledge whatever is present.

Techniques for Resolving Physical Distress: Upon identifying areas of tension, the therapist employs targeted EMDR techniques to facilitate relief. This may involve additional rounds of bilateral stimulation, focusing specifically on the sensations identified during the body scan. The therapist might also integrate other therapeutic interventions, such as guided imagery or mindfulness techniques, to help the client release the physical tension. These methods are selected based on the client's response and comfort level, ensuring a tailored approach to addressing bodily distress.

Deepening the Release: The therapist encourages the client to visualize the tension dissipating or being released from their body. This imaginative process is supported by continued bilateral stimulation, enhancing the client's ability to let go of the residual physical stress. The therapist may also guide the client in incorporating positive beliefs or affirmations related to bodily safety and well-being, reinforcing the connection between physical relaxation and emotional healing.

Reassessing the Body: After working through areas of tension, the client is asked to conduct another scan of their body to assess changes in their physical sensations. This reassessment is vital for recognizing progress and identifying any additional areas that may require attention. It also serves as a reflective practice, allowing the client to experience the tangible benefits of releasing physical manifestations of trauma.

Closing the Phase: The body scan phase concludes with the therapist ensuring that the client feels a sense of calm and physical ease. If any tension remains, the therapist may decide to revisit certain areas in future sessions or employ alternative strategies to support the client's journey towards complete physical and emotional integration.

Throughout this phase, the therapist's role is to provide a safe and supportive environment, guiding the client with patience and empathy. The body scan is not just a technique for identifying physical distress but also an opportunity for clients to reconnect with their bodies, often leading to profound insights and a deeper sense of embodiment. By addressing both the psychological and somatic components of trauma, EMDR therapy fosters a comprehensive healing process, empowering clients to achieve a state of balance and well-being.

2.7: CLOSURE TECHNIQUES FOR CLIENT STABILIZATION

The closure phase is critical in ensuring that clients leave sessions feeling stable and equipped with strategies for managing emotional disturbances that may arise between sessions. This phase acts as a bridge between the intense work of EMDR processing and the client's return to their daily life. It's essential to provide clients with a sense of safety and tools for self-regulation to maintain the progress achieved during the session.

Debriefing is the first step in this phase, where the therapist and client review the session together. This process helps clients integrate their experiences and reinforces their understanding of the progress made. It's an opportunity to validate their feelings and the hard work they've put into their healing journey.

Calming Techniques should be introduced or revisited at this point. Techniques such as deep breathing, visualization of a safe place, or mindfulness exercises can be very effective. These strategies are not only useful in the therapy room but are also invaluable tools for clients to use whenever they feel overwhelmed by distressing emotions or memories outside of sessions.

Creating a Safety Plan is another crucial component. Therapists should work with clients to develop a plan that they can implement if they experience heightened distress or intrusive memories between sessions. This plan might include a list of calming techniques, a reminder of their safe place, and contact information for support networks or crisis services if needed.

Empowering the Client is a fundamental goal of the closure phase. Reinforcing the client's ability to manage their emotional state and reminding them of the progress they've made helps build confidence. It's important to remind clients that they have the tools and skills to face challenges that may arise, reinforcing their sense of agency and resilience.

Scheduling the Next Session provides clients with a clear expectation of their continued path to recovery. It helps to mitigate anxiety about the future by knowing that there is a set time when they will receive further support.

Incorporating these techniques into the closure phase of EMDR therapy ensures that clients leave sessions feeling grounded, empowered, and equipped to handle the emotional challenges that may arise between sessions. It's a crucial step in supporting their overall healing journey and in reinforcing the progress made during therapy.

2.8: REEVALUATION PROCESS IN THERAPY

The reevaluation phase is a critical component of the EMDR therapy process, serving as a mechanism to assess the client's progress and to plan future directions for treatment. This phase allows both the therapist and the client to evaluate the effectiveness of the treatment thus far and to adjust the therapeutic plan as necessary. It is an ongoing process that occurs after the completion of the initial treatment phases and continues throughout the therapeutic relationship to ensure that the therapy is meeting the client's evolving needs.

During reevaluation, therapists revisit the treatment goals established at the outset of therapy to determine the extent to which they have been achieved. This involves a comprehensive review of the client's symptoms, behaviors, and overall functioning. Therapists may use standardized assessment tools or scales to quantify changes in the client's status and to provide an objective measure of progress. Additionally, subjective reports from the client about their experiences, emotional state, and coping strategies are equally valuable in this assessment.

One key aspect of reevaluation is the examination of any remaining distressing memories or symptoms that have not been fully resolved. This may involve identifying new target memories that have emerged as a result of the therapy or reassessing previously targeted memories to ensure that they no longer elicit distress. The therapist and client collaboratively decide whether additional EMDR sessions focusing on these targets are necessary.

Another important consideration during the reevaluation phase is the assessment of the client's current coping mechanisms and emotional regulation strategies. The therapy may have facilitated the development of new skills and resources for managing distress, and it is important to evaluate the effectiveness and sustainability of these strategies. This assessment can guide the therapist in providing further support or interventions to strengthen the client's resilience and coping capacity.

The reevaluation phase also offers an opportunity to address any new challenges or stressors that have arisen in the client's life since the initiation of therapy. Life events, changes in circumstances, or the emergence of new symptoms can all impact the client's well-being and may necessitate adjustments to the treatment plan. This phase ensures that the therapy remains responsive to the client's current needs and circumstances.

In cases where the client has made significant progress and achieved their treatment goals, the reevaluation phase can serve as a transition to discussing the conclusion of therapy or moving towards a maintenance phase of treatment. This might involve spacing sessions further apart or focusing on reinforcing the gains made during therapy to prevent relapse.

Ultimately, the reevaluation phase is a dynamic and collaborative process that underscores the adaptive nature of EMDR therapy. It ensures that treatment is tailored to the client's ongoing needs and progress, facilitating a flexible and responsive approach to trauma recovery. Through regular reevaluation, therapists can provide targeted interventions that address the client's current challenges and support their continued healing and growth.

Chapter 3: Essential Tools for EMDR Therapists

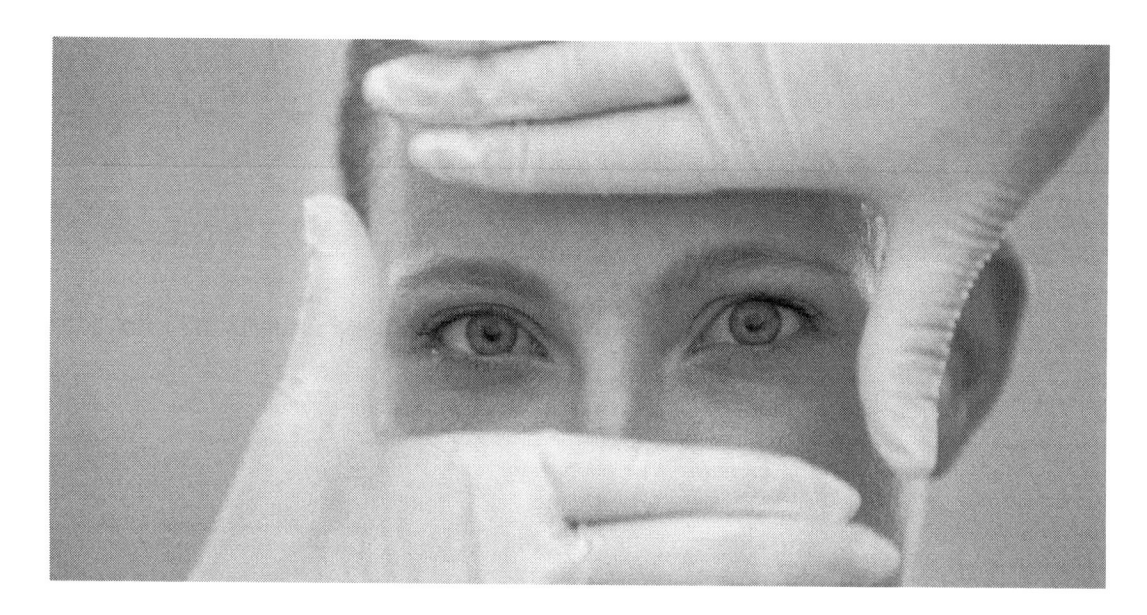

3.1: BUILDING RAPPORT WITH CLIENTS

Establishing a strong therapeutic alliance is paramount in Eye Movement Desensitization and Reprocessing (EMDR) therapy, as it sets the foundation for effective trauma processing. The initial step towards building rapport with clients involves active listening, which signifies to the client that their experiences and feelings are both heard and valued. This approach fosters an environment of trust and safety, critical for clients to feel comfortable sharing their traumatic experiences.

Empathy is another crucial component. Demonstrating genuine empathy through verbal affirmations and non-verbal cues such as nodding and maintaining eye contact helps clients feel understood and supported. This emotional connection encourages clients to engage more openly in the therapeutic process.

Transparency about the EMDR process is essential. Providing clear explanations about what EMDR is, how it works, and what clients can expect during sessions demystifies the process and helps alleviate any anxieties or misconceptions they may have. This clarity empowers clients, allowing them to feel more in control and less apprehensive about embarking on the therapeutic journey.

Setting realistic expectations is also key. Discussing the potential challenges and successes of EMDR therapy helps manage clients' expectations and prepares them for the range of emotions they may experience. It's important to emphasize that while EMDR can be profoundly transformative, progress often requires navigating through difficult memories and emotions.

Consistency in appointments and procedures helps build a reliable framework for therapy. When clients know what to expect at each session, it enhances their sense of security and trust in the therapeutic process. This consistency also reinforces the therapeutic boundaries, creating a safe space for trauma work.

Finally, celebrating milestones, no matter how small, reinforces the therapeutic alliance. Acknowledging progress not only boosts clients' morale but also strengthens their trust in the therapy and the therapist. It's a reminder of the collaborative effort between the therapist and client, and the shared commitment to the client's healing journey.

By integrating these strategies, therapists can build a strong rapport with their clients, which is instrumental in the success of EMDR therapy. A solid therapeutic alliance not only facilitates the trauma processing work but also supports clients in their broader healing journey, contributing to more positive outcomes in therapy.

3.2: SETTING EXPECTATIONS FOR EMDR

Preparing clients for the Eye Movement Desensitization and Reprocessing (EMDR) process involves a nuanced approach that addresses both the logistical and emotional aspects of therapy. It is crucial to set accurate expectations to mitigate any apprehensions and to foster a conducive environment for healing. The initial conversations should aim to demystify the process, providing a clear and straightforward explanation of what EMDR entails and how it differs from traditional talk therapy. This includes discussing the role of bilateral stimulation as a core component of EMDR and its purpose in facilitating the brain's natural healing processes.

Clarifying the timeline of therapy is essential. Clients often come with the hope of immediate relief, so it is important to communicate that while some may experience rapid progress, EMDR therapy is a journey that unfolds over several sessions. The pace of progress is highly individual, depending on the complexity of the trauma and the individual's response to treatment. Emphasize that this does not reflect on their capability or the effectiveness of the therapy but is a natural part of the healing process.

Addressing common misconceptions is another critical step. Clients may have heard myths or inaccuracies about EMDR, such as it being a quick fix that magically erases traumatic memories. It's vital to explain that EMDR does not erase memories but rather changes the way these memories are stored, reducing their distressing impact. This helps set a realistic framework for what EMDR can achieve.

Discussing potential emotional responses during and after sessions helps clients prepare for the range of emotions that can surface. It's important to reassure them that experiencing strong emotions or recalling forgotten memories is a normal part of the healing process. Providing strategies for self-care and emotional regulation between sessions can empower clients, giving them a sense of control over their healing journey.

Emphasizing the importance of safety within the therapeutic relationship is paramount. Assure clients that their well-being is the primary concern and that the therapy will proceed at a pace that feels comfortable for them. This includes the use of grounding techniques and other safety measures to ensure they feel secure throughout the process.

Finally, **encouraging questions and ongoing dialogue** about their experience with EMDR fosters an open and collaborative therapeutic relationship. It allows clients to voice any concerns or confusion they may have, enabling the therapist to address these promptly and effectively. This ongoing communication is key to adjusting the therapy to meet the client's needs and to reinforcing their active role in their healing process.

By setting clear, realistic expectations and addressing common misconceptions, therapists can help clients approach EMDR therapy with an informed and open mindset, ready to engage in the work necessary for healing. This preparation is a fundamental step in building a strong therapeutic alliance and ensuring a positive therapy experience.

3.3: PREPARING CLIENTS FOR EMDR SESSIONS

Building emotional stability and readiness in clients before they engage in Eye Movement Desensitization and Reprocessing (EMDR) sessions is a critical step in the therapeutic process. This preparation ensures that clients are not only willing but also psychologically prepared to face and reprocess traumatic memories. Emotional stability is paramount for clients to effectively handle the intense emotions that may arise during EMDR therapy. Here are specific strategies and considerations for therapists to enhance client readiness:

Educate the Client on Emotional Responses: It is essential to inform clients about the range of emotional responses they may experience during EMDR therapy. Understanding that feelings such as sadness, anger, or even temporary increases in distress are normal can help clients feel more secure. This knowledge empowers them to face their emotions rather than retreat from them.

Develop Emotional Regulation Skills: Before beginning EMDR, clients should have a toolkit of emotional regulation strategies. Techniques such as deep breathing, mindfulness, and visualization can be invaluable. Therapists should work with clients to develop and practice these skills, ensuring they have reliable methods to manage emotional distress both within and outside of therapy sessions.

Establish a Safe Place: Utilizing the concept of a 'safe place' is a common practice in trauma therapy. Encourage clients to identify or create a mental image of a place where they feel completely safe and at peace. This technique can be a crucial grounding tool during sessions when clients are confronted with distressing memories.

Incremental Exposure to Traumatic Material: To build tolerance for distressing emotions and memories, therapists might initially expose clients to less distressing material. This gradual approach helps clients build confidence in their ability to handle emotional distress, making them more prepared for reprocessing more challenging traumatic memories.

Reinforce the Therapeutic Alliance: The strength of the therapeutic relationship cannot be overstated in its importance for client readiness. Clients who feel a strong, trusting bond with their therapist are more likely to feel safe exploring and reprocessing traumatic memories. Regular check-ins about the client's feelings towards therapy and any concerns they have can strengthen this alliance.

Use of Grounding Techniques: Grounding techniques can help clients maintain a connection to the present moment, providing an anchor to reality when memories become overwhelming. Techniques may include tactile exercises, such as holding a smooth stone, or auditory cues, like listening to calming music. These strategies can help prevent dissociation and ensure clients remain grounded during sessions.

Pre-Session Check-Ins: Before each EMDR session, conduct a brief check-in with the client to assess their current emotional state and readiness to proceed. This can help identify any immediate concerns that need to be addressed and ensure the client feels prepared to engage in the session's work.

Client Autonomy in the Process: Empowering clients by involving them in decisions about the pacing and direction of therapy can significantly enhance their readiness. When clients feel they have a say in their treatment, they are more likely to engage actively and feel prepared for the challenges of EMDR.

By incorporating these strategies, therapists can help clients build the emotional stability and readiness necessary for effective trauma reprocessing. This preparation is not only about making clients ready for EMDR but also about empowering them to engage in the therapeutic process with confidence and resilience.

Part 2: Treating Trauma with EMDR

Chapter 4: Standard Protocols for PTSD

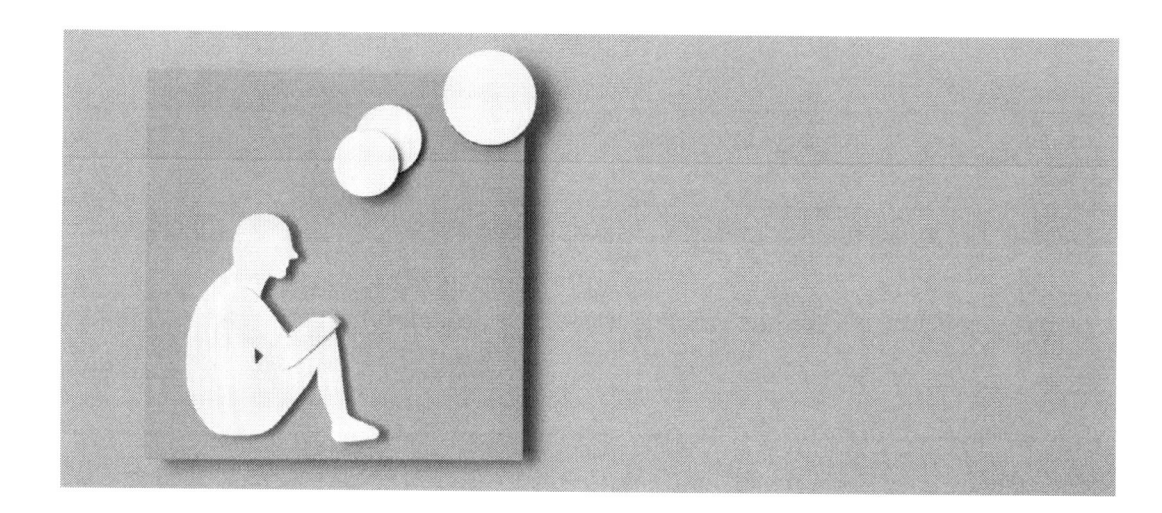

4.1: Selecting Trauma Targets

Selecting the appropriate trauma targets for reprocessing is a critical step in the Eye Movement Desensitization and Reprocessing (EMDR) therapy process. This decision-making process involves a thorough assessment of the client's history and the identification of specific memories that contribute to their current symptoms. The aim is to prioritize these memories based on their intensity and the level of disturbance they cause, facilitating a structured approach to therapy that maximizes therapeutic outcomes.

Identifying Key Memories: Begin by engaging the client in a detailed exploration of their life history, focusing on traumatic events and distressing experiences. This exploration will help in pinpointing specific incidents that are pivotal to the client's psychological distress. It's essential to assess the emotional charge and disturbance level associated with each memory, utilizing tools such as the Subjective Units of Disturbance Scale (SUDS) to quantify the client's emotional response.

Prioritizing Memories for Reprocessing: Once key memories have been identified, the next step is to prioritize them for reprocessing. Prioritization should take into account the client's current level of stability, the potential for re-traumatization, and the therapeutic goals established during the treatment planning phase. It's often advisable to start with memories that are less distressing, gradually working up to more challenging ones as the client builds resilience and coping mechanisms.

Considering the Client's Readiness: Assessing the client's readiness for reprocessing is paramount. Ensure that the client has developed sufficient coping strategies and is in a stable enough state to handle the emotional intensity of reprocessing traumatic memories. This assessment should be an ongoing process, with regular check-ins to adjust the treatment plan as needed.

Addressing Complex Trauma: In cases of complex trauma, where multiple interrelated traumatic memories exist, it may be necessary to adopt a more nuanced approach. This could involve identifying themes or patterns that link different memories, focusing on these interconnected aspects to facilitate a more comprehensive resolution of trauma.

Collaborative Decision Making: The process of selecting and prioritizing trauma targets should be a collaborative effort between the therapist and the client. This collaborative approach ensures that the client feels a sense of control and agency over their treatment process, which is crucial for building trust and fostering a positive therapeutic relationship.

Flexibility in the Reprocessing Sequence: While a structured approach to selecting trauma targets is beneficial, it's also important to remain flexible. The therapy process is dynamic, and new memories or insights may emerge that necessitate adjustments to the treatment plan. Being adaptable allows for the incorporation of these new elements, ensuring that the therapy remains responsive to the client's evolving needs.

In summary, the careful selection and prioritization of trauma targets are foundational aspects of effective EMDR therapy. By taking a structured yet flexible approach, therapists can help clients navigate the path to recovery with greater efficacy, ensuring that each step in the therapy process contributes to their overall healing and well-being.

4.2: MANAGING FLASHBACKS WITH EMDR

Eye Movement Desensitization and Reprocessing (EMDR) therapy offers a powerful approach to managing flashbacks and intrusive thoughts, core symptoms that often plague individuals with Post-Traumatic Stress Disorder (PTSD). These symptoms can be intensely disruptive, hijacking a person's sense of safety and control. EMDR addresses these challenges by facilitating the processing of traumatic memories, thus reducing their lingering power.

The mechanism at the heart of EMDR's effectiveness lies in its unique use of bilateral stimulation, typically through guided eye movements, auditory tones, or tactile taps. This stimulation is believed to mimic the psychological state associated with Rapid Eye Movement (REM) sleep, promoting an accelerated information processing by the brain. During this state, individuals can access and reprocess traumatic memories in a way that diminishes their emotional intensity.

Bilateral stimulation serves as a distraction technique, helping individuals maintain a dual focus of attention. This dual focus allows them to remain grounded in the present while revisiting past traumas. The process transforms the memory's status from a current threat to a historical event, thereby reducing its capacity to trigger flashbacks and intrusive thoughts.

Desensitization is a critical phase in EMDR where the therapist guides the client to target the traumatic memory while simultaneously engaging in bilateral stimulation. This phase aims to decrease the emotional charge associated with the memory. As desensitization progresses, clients often report a significant reduction in the vividness and emotional impact of the memory, leading to fewer flashbacks and intrusive thoughts.

Installation of positive beliefs is another essential component of EMDR. After the charge of the traumatic memory has been reduced, therapists help clients anchor positive cognitions about themselves in relation to the memory. For instance, shifting from "I am in danger" to "I am safe now" can profoundly alter how individuals perceive themselves and their capacity to navigate the world safely.

Body scanning further aids in identifying and addressing any residual somatic distress linked to the traumatic memory. Clients are encouraged to notice physical sensations while thinking of the event and the installed positive belief. This process helps in releasing any stored tension related to the trauma, contributing to a comprehensive resolution of the symptoms.

The **Closure** phase ensures that clients are returned to a state of equilibrium at the end of each session, equipped with techniques for emotional regulation to manage any residual disturbances. This phase is crucial for maintaining stability and preventing a spike in symptoms between sessions.

Reevaluation, occurring in subsequent sessions, assesses the effectiveness of the treatment in reducing symptoms and improving the client's quality of life. This continuous monitoring allows for adjustments in the therapeutic approach, ensuring that the therapy addresses all aspects of the client's PTSD symptoms.

EMDR therapy stands out for its structured yet flexible approach to treating PTSD. By directly targeting the memories that fuel flashbacks and intrusive thoughts, EMDR offers a path to recovery that is both efficient and enduring. Its effectiveness is not just in managing symptoms but in fundamentally altering the way traumatic memories are stored and experienced, paving the way for a renewed sense of personal power and emotional freedom.

4.3: SINGLE-EVENT VS. COMPLEX TRAUMA APPROACHES

When addressing single-event trauma versus complex trauma, therapists are faced with distinct challenges and considerations. Single-event trauma, often resulting from a one-time occurrence such as an accident, natural disaster, or violent attack, typically involves a clear, identifiable memory. In contrast, complex trauma stems from repeated or prolonged exposure to highly stressful situations, such as abuse, neglect, or living in a war-torn region, leading to multifaceted psychological impacts.

Single-Event Trauma: Approach and Techniques

For individuals experiencing single-event trauma, the therapeutic focus is on processing the traumatic incident to reduce its power and integrating the experience into their life narrative. The Adaptive Information Processing (AIP) model suggests that trauma disrupts the normal processing of information, leaving the memory unassimilated and causing symptoms of PTSD. In these cases, EMDR therapy aims to facilitate the processing of the specific memory, allowing it to be stored adaptively in the brain. This often involves fewer sessions than complex trauma, as there is typically a single focal point for treatment. Techniques include:

1. **Targeting the Traumatic Memory**: Identifying the memory of the single event and using EMDR protocols to desensitize the client to the emotional and physiological responses associated with it.

2. **Installation of Positive Cognitions**: Replacing negative beliefs that have arisen from the trauma ("I am in danger") with positive ones ("I am safe now").

3. **Body Scanning**: To resolve any residual somatic symptoms linked to the traumatic memory.

Complex Trauma: Approach and Techniques

Complex trauma requires a more layered approach due to the interwoven nature of traumatic memories and the potential for significant dissociation and emotional dysregulation. The treatment often extends over a longer period, addressing the multiple aspects of the trauma and its pervasive impact on the individual's life. Key strategies include:

1. **Stabilization**: Before processing any traumatic memories, it's crucial to ensure the client has strong coping mechanisms and a sense of safety. This may involve grounding techniques, establishing a therapeutic alliance, and teaching emotional regulation skills.

2. **Phased Reprocessing**: Given the complexity and number of traumatic memories, a phased approach is often necessary. This begins with less distressing memories or those most impacting current functioning, gradually moving to more challenging ones.

3. **Working with Dissociation**: Complex trauma often involves dissociative symptoms. Therapists must be adept at recognizing and managing dissociation, ensuring the client remains grounded and present during sessions.

4. **Integration and Reconnection**: The goal is to help the client integrate the processed memories into a coherent narrative and reconnect with previously avoided aspects of life, fostering a sense of identity beyond the trauma.

Differences in Treatment Planning and Outcomes

The primary difference in treating single-event versus complex trauma lies in the scope and depth of therapeutic intervention required. Single-event trauma, with its focused target for reprocessing, may lead to quicker symptom resolution. Conversely, complex trauma demands a comprehensive, often multi-modal approach that addresses the layers of trauma and their pervasive effects on the person's mental health, relationships, and sense of self.

In both cases, the therapist's sensitivity to the client's readiness, pacing of therapy, and ongoing assessment of therapeutic needs are paramount. The ultimate aim is not only the reduction of symptoms but the enhancement of resilience, empowerment, and post-traumatic growth, allowing individuals to move beyond their traumatic experiences towards a more fulfilling life.

Chapter 5: Dissociation Challenges and Solutions

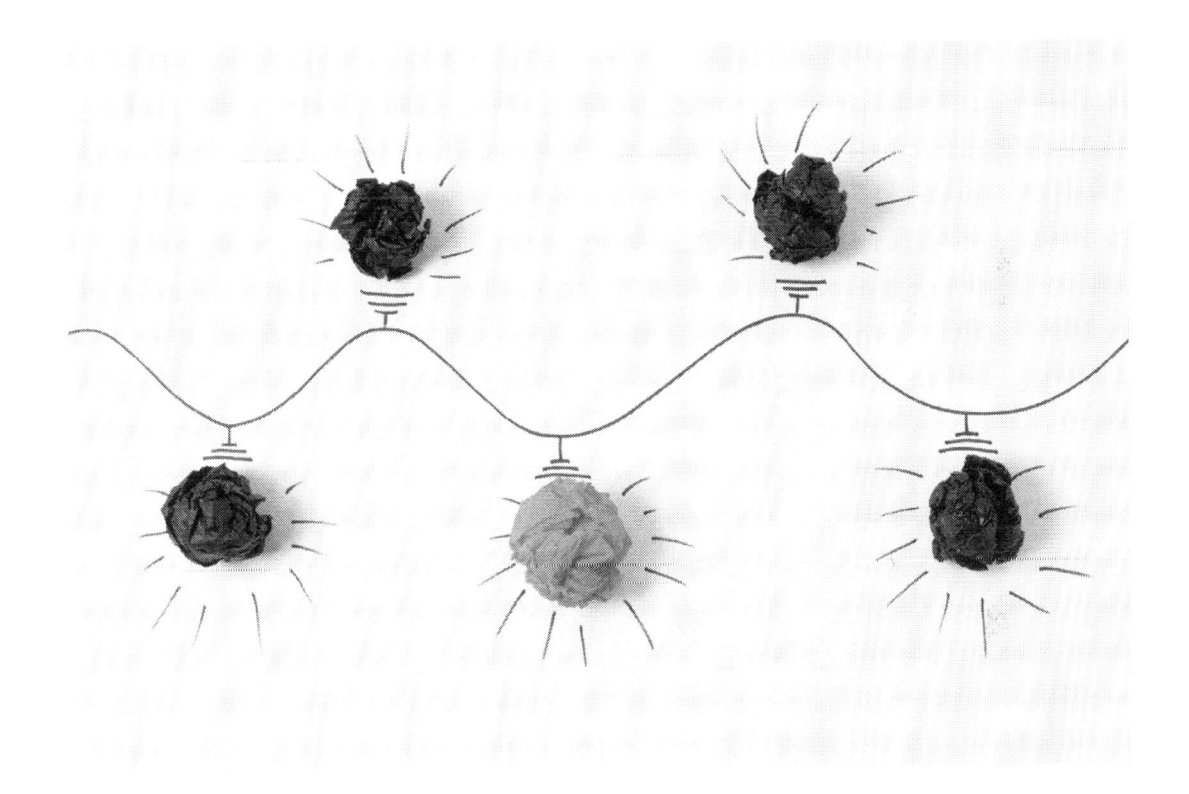

5.1: UNDERSTANDING DISSOCIATION IN EMDR THERAPY

Dissociation is a psychological phenomenon where an individual may feel disconnected from their thoughts, feelings, memories, or sense of identity. In the context of Eye Movement Desensitization and Reprocessing (EMDR) therapy, understanding dissociation is crucial, as it significantly impacts the processing of traumatic memories. Dissociation can serve as a defense mechanism against overwhelming trauma, allowing an individual to endure distressing experiences by detaching from them emotionally or cognitively. However, this detachment can hinder the effective processing of traumatic memories, making it a critical factor for therapists to address in treatment.

The Effects of Dissociation on Trauma Processing

1. **Impedes Emotional Processing**: Dissociation can block the emotional processing necessary for the adaptive resolution of traumatic memories. When a client dissociates, they may not fully engage with the memory or the associated emotions, limiting the effectiveness of EMDR therapy.

2. **Disrupts Memory Consolidation**: The fragmented nature of dissociative experiences can lead to disjointed and disorganized memories. This fragmentation complicates the task of identifying and targeting specific memories for reprocessing in EMDR therapy.

3. **Affects Client Safety**: Clients who dissociate frequently may struggle to remain grounded in the present during EMDR sessions. This poses a challenge in maintaining a safe therapeutic environment where the client can process trauma without becoming overwhelmed.

4. **Hinders Therapeutic Alliance**: The presence of dissociation can make it difficult for therapists to establish and maintain a strong therapeutic alliance. Clients who dissociate might appear distant or unengaged, which can be misinterpreted as resistance to therapy.

Strategies for Managing Dissociation in EMDR Therapy

- **Preparation and Stabilization**: Before proceeding with trauma reprocessing, it is essential to ensure that the client has strategies in place to manage dissociation. Techniques such as grounding exercises can help clients maintain a connection to the present moment.

- **Safe Place Exercise**: Establishing a 'safe place'—a mental imagery exercise where the client imagines a secure and comforting space—can be particularly beneficial for clients prone to dissociation. This exercise can provide a quick way for clients to re-ground themselves if they begin to dissociate during a session.

- **Pacing the Therapy**: For clients who experience significant dissociation, it may be necessary to pace the therapy more slowly. This approach allows for the gradual processing of traumatic material in a way that does not overwhelm the client's capacity to stay present.

- **Integration of Dissociative Parts**: In cases of severe dissociation, such as Dissociative Identity Disorder (DID), therapy may involve working with different dissociative parts of the client. Recognizing and addressing these parts can facilitate a more comprehensive processing of trauma.

- **Continuous Monitoring and Adjustment**: Therapists should continuously monitor the client's level of dissociation throughout the EMDR process. Adjustments to the therapy plan may be required to ensure that the client remains safe and engaged.

In summary, dissociation presents unique challenges in the treatment of trauma with EMDR therapy. By understanding the nature of dissociation and its impact on trauma processing, therapists can employ specific strategies to mitigate these challenges. This involves careful preparation, pacing, and monitoring of the client, with an emphasis on safety and engagement. Through these tailored approaches, therapists can enhance the effectiveness of EMDR therapy for clients who experience dissociation, facilitating their journey towards healing and recovery.

5.2 Grounding Techniques for Stabilization

Objective: To utilize grounding techniques that enhance the sense of safety and reduce dissociative episodes during EMDR sessions, facilitating a more stable therapeutic process.

Step-by-step instructions:

1. **Begin with a Safe Space Visualization:**

    - Ask the client to close their eyes (if comfortable) and visualize a place where they feel completely safe and at ease. This could be a real or imaginary place.

    - Guide them to notice the details of this safe space—the colors, sounds, smells, and textures.

    - Encourage them to stay in this visualization for a few minutes, deepening their sense of safety and relaxation.

2. **5-4-3-2-1 Technique:**

    - Instruct the client to name 5 things they can see in the room.

    - Ask them to identify 4 sounds they can hear at the moment.

    - Have them touch 3 objects and describe the texture and temperature.

    - Request them to identify 2 different smells, or if that's not applicable, to name 2 favorite scents they remember.

    - Finally, ask them to name 1 thing they can taste or like to taste.

3. **Deep Breathing with a Focus on Exhalation:**

    - Guide the client to take slow, deep breaths, focusing particularly on making the exhalation longer than the inhalation.

    - This can be facilitated by counting to 4 while inhaling and to 6 or 8 while exhaling, helping to activate the parasympathetic nervous system and promote a sense of calm.

4. **Tactile Anchoring:**

- Provide the client with a small object, such as a stone, a soft ball, or a textured fabric.

- Encourage them to hold the object in their hand, focusing on its weight, texture, and temperature as a means to stay present and grounded.

5. **Progressive Muscle Relaxation:**

- Guide the client through a progressive muscle relaxation exercise, starting from the toes and moving up to the head.

- Instruct them to tense each muscle group for a few seconds and then release, noticing the contrast between tension and relaxation.

6. **Utilize Bilateral Stimulation as a Grounding Tool:**

- While the client is seated, ask them to place their feet flat on the floor and notice the contact with the ground.

- Introduce a gentle bilateral stimulation, such as tapping knees alternately, to help maintain present-moment awareness and reduce dissociation.

7. **Mindful Observation of the Environment:**

- Invite the client to look around the room and describe their surroundings in detail, including colors, shapes, and any movement.

- This practice helps redirect attention from internal distress to external reality, reinforcing a sense of safety and presence.

8. **Encourage Journaling Post-Session:**

- Suggest that the client keeps a journal to document their experiences with grounding techniques during and between sessions.

- This can help them identify which strategies are most effective for them and encourage active participation in their healing process.

Each of these steps can be tailored to the individual needs and preferences of the client, ensuring that the grounding techniques provide meaningful support in their journey through EMDR therapy.

5.3: Identifying and Addressing Dissociative Subsystems

When addressing dissociative subsystems within the context of Eye Movement Desensitization and Reprocessing (EMDR), it is essential to understand that these fragmented identities or parts have likely developed as a protective mechanism in response to trauma. The primary goal is to facilitate communication and integration among these parts to achieve a more cohesive sense of self for the client. The following strategies are pivotal in working with dissociative subsystems:

1. **Establishing Safety and Trust:** Before any direct engagement with dissociative parts, ensure that a strong therapeutic alliance is in place. This foundation of safety and trust is critical for clients to feel secure enough to explore and work with their fragmented identities.

2. **Identifying Dissociative Parts:** Utilize techniques that allow clients to identify and acknowledge the existence of different parts. This may involve structured dissociation questionnaires, creative expression, or guided imagery exercises designed to gently surface these parts to consciousness.

3. **Understanding the Function of Each Part:** Each dissociative part serves a specific role or function, often related to coping with or escaping from traumatic experiences. Engage clients in a dialogue (either directly or through imaginative exercises) to uncover the purpose and origins of each part.

4. **Promoting Internal Communication:** Encourage and facilitate communication between dissociative parts. This can be approached through internal family systems (IFS) therapy techniques, where parts are invited to express their concerns, needs, and desires in a safe and structured manner.

5. **Gradual Exposure to Trauma Processing:** With dissociative clients, a cautious and gradual approach to trauma processing is necessary. Begin with less distressing memories or parts, slowly building the client's capacity for processing more challenging material. This stepwise approach helps prevent overwhelming the system and reinforces the client's sense of control and safety.

6. Integration Work: Integration does not necessarily mean merging all parts into a single identity. Instead, focus on fostering cooperation and harmony among parts, helping the client develop a more unified and resilient sense of self. Techniques may include narrative therapy, where parts are encouraged to share their stories and find common ground.

7. Continuous Assessment and Flexibility: Be prepared to adjust strategies based on the client's responses and the dynamics between parts. Continuous assessment allows for the tailoring of interventions to meet the unique needs and pacing of each client.

8. Reinforcing the Client's Present Safety: Throughout the process, it's crucial to reinforce the client's sense of safety in the present moment. Grounding techniques and reminders of the here-and-now help mitigate the risk of re-traumatization and ensure that exploration of dissociative parts occurs within a secure therapeutic context.

9. Collaborative Goal Setting: Work collaboratively with the client and their parts to establish goals for therapy. This inclusive approach ensures that all parts feel heard and valued, contributing to a more integrated and cohesive treatment process.

10. Encouraging Self-Compassion: Foster an attitude of self-compassion within the client towards all their parts. Recognizing that each part has played a role in the individual's survival and coping can promote acceptance and understanding within the internal system.

By employing these strategies, therapists can effectively navigate the complexities of dissociative subsystems within EMDR therapy. The focus on safety, gradual exposure, integration, and collaboration respects the client's experiences and promotes healing in a structured yet flexible framework.

Part 3:
Adapting EMDR for Complex Cases

Chapter 6: Tailoring EMDR for Complex PTSD

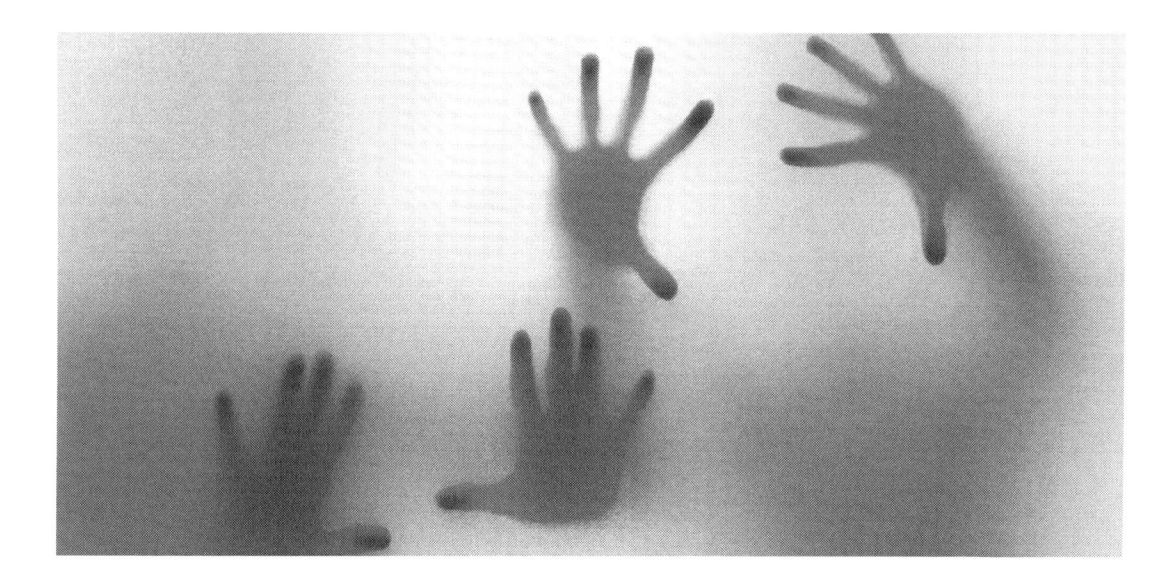

6.1: RECOGNIZING SIGNS OF COMPLEX TRAUMA

Identifying complex PTSD (C-PTSD) requires a nuanced understanding of its symptoms, which often overlap with those of other mental health conditions yet are distinguished by their roots in prolonged, repeated trauma. Unlike PTSD, which might develop after a single traumatic event, C-PTSD emerges from enduring exposure to traumatic situations such as long-term abuse, captivity, or exposure to war zones. To differentiate complex PTSD from other disorders, therapists should look for a constellation of symptoms that extend beyond the typical PTSD symptomatology.

Key Symptoms of Complex PTSD include:

- **Persistent Emotional Dysregulation**: Unlike the more episodic emotional reactions seen in PTSD, individuals with C-PTSD may experience constant difficulties with emotional regulation, manifesting as chronic anger, sadness, or suicidal thoughts.

- **Disturbances in Self-Perception**: People suffering from C-PTSD often struggle with feelings of shame, guilt, or a persistent sense of being completely different from others. This might include a deep feeling of worthlessness or a preoccupation with being perceived as evil or bad.

- **Difficulties in Relationships**: Those with complex PTSD may find it hard to form or maintain relationships due to mistrust, a constant search for a rescuer, or a tendency to re-enact the trauma with others.

- **Preoccupation with the Perpetrator**: This can range from preoccupations with revenge to an idealization of the perpetrator or a preoccupation with the relationship.

- **Loss of Systems of Meanings**: Individuals may experience a loss of faith or a profound sense of hopelessness about the world and their place in it, which is more pervasive than the sense of threat or mistrust seen in PTSD.

- **Somatic Symptoms**: Chronic pain or health issues without a clear medical diagnosis can also be a sign of C-PTSD, as the trauma is often held within the body.

Differentiation from Other Conditions involves:

- **Assessing the Duration and Nature of Trauma**: Understanding the timeline and type of trauma experienced by the individual can help differentiate C-PTSD from PTSD, which is often linked to a single event or a series of discrete events.

- **Evaluating Interpersonal Relationship Patterns**: The complex interplay of symptoms in C-PTSD often leads to more pronounced difficulties in interpersonal relationships than those seen in PTSD or other anxiety disorders.

- **Observing Emotional Responses**: The chronic, pervasive nature of emotional dysregulation in C-PTSD, including feelings of shame and guilt, can help distinguish it from the more episodic or situation-specific responses seen in PTSD.

- **Understanding Self-Perception**: The distorted self-perception and identity issues are more characteristic of C-PTSD than PTSD, where negative beliefs about oneself are usually related to the traumatic event rather than a pervasive sense of worthlessness.

- **Physical Health**: Chronic, unexplained physical complaints, along with a history of trauma, may also point towards C-PTSD.

In practice, the differentiation between complex PTSD and other mental health conditions requires a comprehensive assessment, including a detailed trauma history and an understanding of the individual's symptomatology over time. Therapists should also be mindful of the potential for comorbid conditions, such as depression and anxiety disorders, which can complicate the clinical picture. Recognizing the signs of complex PTSD is the first step in providing effective treatment and support for those affected by this profound and debilitating condition.

6.2: ADJUSTING PROTOCOLS FOR SAFETY AND TOLERANCE

Adjusting protocols for safety and tolerance is pivotal in ensuring client stability during reprocessing sessions, especially when dealing with complex PTSD. The primary goal is to modulate the intensity of the therapeutic process to prevent overwhelming the client while facilitating effective trauma processing. Here are several strategies to achieve this balance:

1. **Slow Pacing**: Introduce a slower pace of therapy, allowing more time for the client to process each memory or trauma aspect. This approach helps in preventing the client from becoming overwhelmed and ensures a sense of control throughout the process.

2. **Interweaving Techniques**: Utilize interweaving techniques to provide relief and perspective when clients become stuck or overly distressed. This can involve temporarily shifting focus away from the traumatic memory to a neutral or positive thought, thereby reducing immediate distress.

3. **Resource Development and Installation (RDI)**: Before delving into trauma reprocessing, work on developing and reinforcing internal resources. Techniques such as creating a 'safe place' or empowering the client with a sense of protection can enhance their tolerance for distressing memories.

4. **Titration**: Break down the processing of traumatic memories into smaller, more manageable parts. This approach, known as titration, avoids overwhelming the client's capacity to process the trauma by introducing it in smaller doses.

5. **Frequent Check-ins**: Regularly check in with the client about their comfort level and sense of safety. This practice helps in making necessary adjustments in real-time and reinforces the collaborative nature of the therapeutic process.

6. **Use of Bilateral Stimulation (BLS)**: Adjust the intensity and type of bilateral stimulation based on the client's response. Some clients may find certain types of BLS more tolerable than others, and the intensity can be varied to match the client's current state.

7. **Flexible Use of Phases**: Be flexible in moving between different phases of EMDR therapy based on the client's needs. It may be necessary to return to earlier phases of therapy, such as preparation or stabilization, if the client experiences significant distress.

8. **Incorporating Mindfulness and Relaxation Techniques**: Teach clients mindfulness and relaxation techniques that they can use during and outside of sessions. These skills can help manage arousal levels and increase distress tolerance.

9. **Adjusting Session Length and Frequency**: Tailor the length and frequency of sessions to the client's capacity to tolerate and process trauma. Some clients may benefit from shorter, more frequent sessions, while others may need longer intervals between sessions for processing and recovery.

10. **Safety Planning**: Develop a clear safety plan that the client can follow outside of sessions. This should include coping strategies, a list of supportive contacts, and steps to take if they feel overwhelmed.

By employing these strategies, therapists can create a therapeutic environment that maximizes safety and tolerance for clients with complex PTSD. This careful adjustment of protocols ensures that the reprocessing of traumatic memories occurs within the client's window of tolerance, facilitating healing while minimizing the risk of re-traumatization.

Chapter 7: Navigating Therapy Blocks

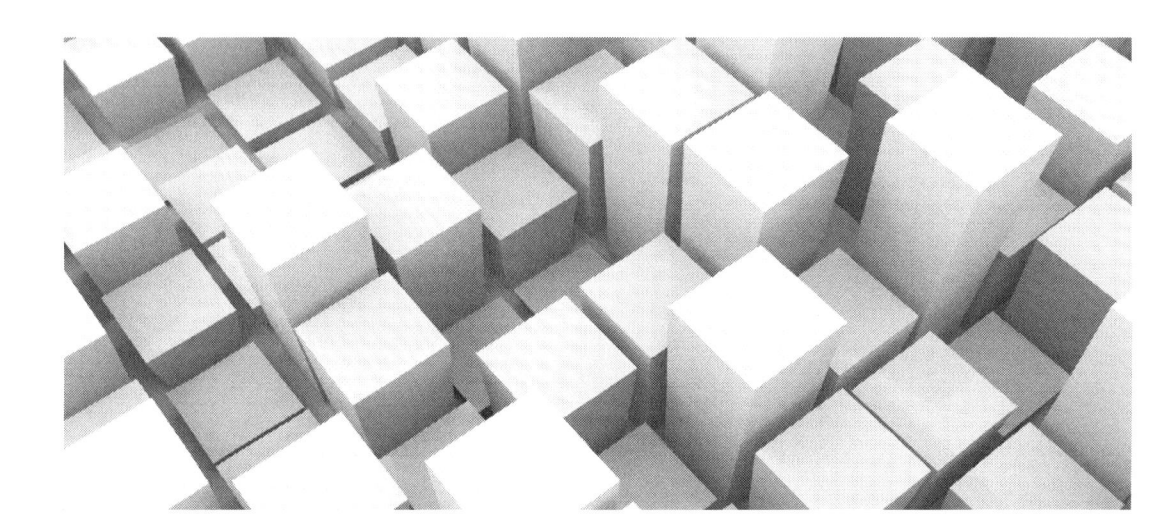

7.1: Identifying and Resolving Cognitive Blocks

Identifying and resolving cognitive and emotional blocks is a critical aspect of EMDR therapy, as these obstacles can significantly hinder the therapeutic process and the client's journey towards healing. Cognitive and emotional blocks often manifest as resistance, which may be rooted in fear, mistrust, or a lack of readiness to confront traumatic memories. To effectively address these challenges, therapists must employ a variety of strategies tailored to the individual needs of their clients.

Understanding the Nature of Resistance

Resistance in therapy can take many forms, from overt refusal to engage in the process to more subtle forms of avoidance or minimization of trauma. It's essential to recognize that resistance is a normal and protective response, serving as a defense mechanism to safeguard the individual from perceived threats or discomfort. Acknowledging and validating the client's experience of resistance is the first step in addressing it.

Strategies for Uncovering Resistance

1. **Active Listening and Empathetic Engagement**: Create a safe and non-judgmental space for clients to express their fears and concerns. Active listening and empathetic engagement can help clients feel understood and supported, reducing the intensity of resistance.

2. **Psychoeducation**: Educate clients about the nature of resistance and its role in the healing process. Understanding that resistance is a common and natural response can help demystify their experience and encourage openness to the therapeutic process.

3. **Identifying Underlying Fears**: Work collaboratively with the client to explore the underlying fears or beliefs contributing to resistance. This may involve discussing past experiences of helplessness, betrayal, or loss that may be influencing their current state.

Techniques for Resolving Cognitive and Emotional Blocks

1. **Gradual Exposure**: Introduce the concept of gradual exposure to traumatic memories, emphasizing the control the client has over the pace and intensity of the process. This approach can help mitigate fear and build trust in the therapeutic relationship.

2. **Resource Development and Installation (RDI)**: Before addressing traumatic memories directly, focus on developing internal resources such as a safe place or protective figures. These resources can provide emotional support and resilience, making it easier to confront and process difficult memories.

3. **Cognitive Restructuring**: Assist clients in identifying and challenging negative beliefs or self-perceptions that may be reinforcing resistance. Cognitive restructuring aims to replace these maladaptive thoughts with more adaptive and empowering beliefs.

4. **Mindfulness and Relaxation Techniques**: Teach clients mindfulness and relaxation techniques to manage emotional and physiological responses to distressing memories. These skills can enhance emotional regulation and reduce the intensity of resistance.

5. **Somatic Experiencing**: Encourage clients to pay attention to bodily sensations and responses as a way to access and process unresolved trauma. Somatic experiencing can help bypass cognitive resistance by focusing on the physical aspects of trauma.

6. **Interweaving Positive Memories**: Integrate positive memories or experiences into the EMDR process to counterbalance the distress associated with traumatic memories. This technique can help reinforce a sense of safety and positivity, reducing resistance.

7. **Collaborative Goal Setting**: Involve clients in setting realistic and achievable goals for therapy. Collaborative goal setting fosters a sense of agency and investment in the therapeutic process, which can help overcome resistance.

By employing these strategies, therapists can effectively navigate cognitive and emotional blocks, facilitating a more productive and healing EMDR experience for their clients. It's important to approach resistance with patience, understanding, and flexibility, adapting interventions to meet the unique needs and readiness of each individual.

7.2: STRATEGIES FOR OVERCOMING RESISTANCE

In addressing resistance within the therapeutic context, particularly in the realm of EMDR, it is paramount to adopt a multifaceted approach that respects the client's pace while methodically guiding them towards engagement. Resistance, often a manifestation of the client's attempt to protect themselves from perceived threats or discomfort, requires a nuanced understanding and strategic interventions to foster a conducive environment for progress. The following strategies are instrumental in overcoming resistance, thereby re-establishing progress and building client trust:

1. **Validation and Normalization**: Begin by validating the client's feelings of resistance, acknowledging it as a natural and understandable response given their history and current circumstances. Normalize their experience by assuring them that resistance is a common reaction in the therapeutic process, which can significantly reduce the client's sense of isolation and stigma.

2. **Therapeutic Alliance Strengthening**: Emphasize the development of a strong therapeutic alliance as a cornerstone for overcoming resistance. This involves demonstrating empathy, consistency, and unconditional positive regard. A strong alliance provides the safety net required for clients to explore and eventually work through their resistance.

3. **Motivational Interviewing Techniques**: Utilize motivational interviewing techniques to explore the ambivalence that often underlies resistance. This approach helps clients articulate their own motivations for change in a non-confrontational manner, thereby increasing their readiness to engage in the therapeutic work.

4. **Incremental Exposure**: Gradually expose clients to the concepts and processes of EMDR, starting with less threatening aspects before progressing to more challenging areas. This scaffolded approach helps clients build confidence in their ability to engage with the therapy and manage their responses.

5. **Psychoeducation**: Provide clients with information about the nature of trauma, the rationale behind EMDR, and how it can help them. Understanding

the science behind their experiences and the therapy can demystify the process, reduce fears, and motivate engagement.

6. **Flexible Protocol Adaptation**: Show flexibility in adapting EMDR protocols to meet the client's unique needs and levels of resistance. This may involve spending more time in the preparation phase, adjusting the pace of sessions, or modifying the intensity of bilateral stimulation.

7. **Client Empowerment**: Empower clients by involving them in decision-making processes throughout therapy. Offering choices about which memories to work on, when to take breaks, and other aspects of their treatment can enhance their sense of control and reduce resistance.

8. **Focus on Resources**: Prioritize resource development and installation (RDI) to ensure clients have robust internal coping mechanisms and a sense of safety before proceeding with trauma processing. This focus on strengths and resilience can mitigate resistance by equipping clients with the tools they need to face distressing material.

9. **Reframing Resistance**: Help clients reframe their resistance as a sign of strength and a survival mechanism. This positive reframe can transform resistance from a barrier into a resource that can be harnessed to foster resilience and healing.

10. **Addressing Past Therapy Experiences**: For clients with previous negative therapy experiences, it's crucial to acknowledge and work through these past disappointments. Understanding their history can provide insights into the origins of their resistance and inform strategies to prevent repetition of past therapeutic ruptures.

11. **Consistent Review and Goal Adjustment**: Regularly review therapy goals with the client to ensure they remain relevant and aligned with the client's evolving needs and circumstances. Adjusting goals as necessary can maintain engagement and motivation, reducing resistance.

12. **Use of Imagery and Metaphor**: Employ imagery and metaphor to help clients conceptualize their resistance and the therapeutic process in more

abstract terms. This can provide a new perspective and facilitate a deeper understanding of their experiences and behaviors.

By integrating these strategies, therapists can effectively address and navigate resistance in EMDR therapy. It is through understanding, patience, and strategic intervention that progress can be re-established and the therapeutic alliance strengthened, paving the way for meaningful change and healing.

Chapter 8: EMDR and Comorbid Conditions

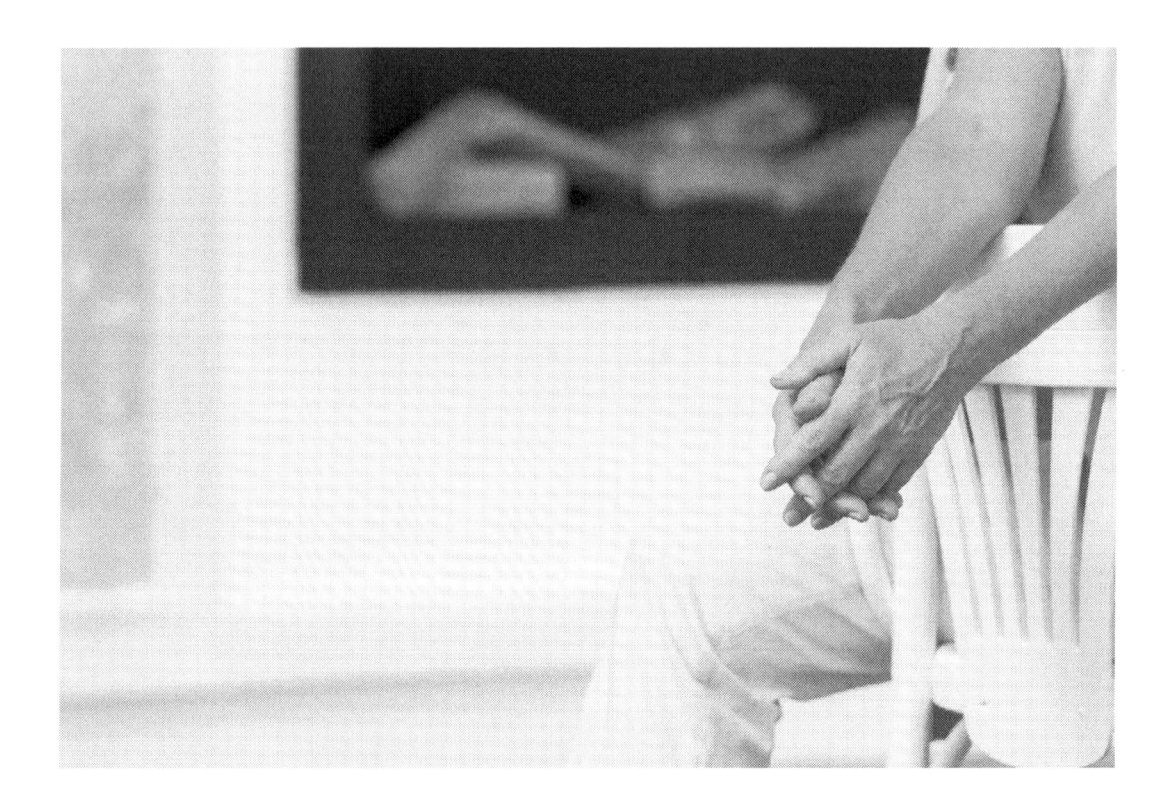

8.1: Working with Anxiety Disorders

Adapting Eye Movement Desensitization and Reprocessing (EMDR) protocols to effectively address symptoms of generalized anxiety and phobias involves a nuanced understanding of these conditions and their impact on individuals. Anxiety disorders, characterized by excessive fear, worry, and a variety of physical symptoms, can significantly impair daily functioning. Phobias, a type of anxiety disorder, involve an intense and irrational fear of specific situations, objects, or activities. The application of EMDR in treating these conditions focuses on desensitizing the client to the sources of fear and reprocessing the underlying memories that contribute to the anxiety response.

Initial Assessment and Target Identification: Begin with a thorough assessment to understand the client's anxiety or phobia in detail. This includes identifying specific triggers, the intensity of the response, and any underlying memories associated with the onset of the disorder. The Subjective Units of Disturbance Scale (SUDS) can be useful in quantifying the client's level of distress related to these triggers.

Preparation Phase Adaptations: Given the heightened sensitivity of clients with anxiety disorders, the preparation phase should emphasize building a strong therapeutic alliance and ensuring the client feels safe and understood. Techniques for managing acute anxiety, such as deep breathing and mindfulness, should be introduced early on. Establishing a 'safe place' imagery is particularly crucial for clients with phobias, providing them with a mental refuge they can access during or outside of therapy sessions.

Desensitization with Gradual Exposure: For clients with phobias, gradual exposure to the feared object or situation can be integrated within the EMDR protocol. Starting with less threatening aspects of the phobia and progressively moving towards more distressing stimuli allows for a controlled desensitization process. This approach should be carefully paced according to the client's tolerance levels to avoid overwhelming them.

Cognitive Interweaves for Challenging Beliefs: Anxiety often involves maladaptive beliefs about the danger posed by certain situations or the individual's ability to cope with them. Cognitive interweaves, which are strategic interventions used during the desensitization phase, can help challenge and reframe these beliefs. For instance, if a client believes they will be unable to survive an encounter with the phobic stimulus, the therapist might interweave questions or statements that highlight the client's past successes in coping with difficult situations.

Resourcing for Emotional Regulation: Clients with generalized anxiety may benefit from enhanced resourcing before proceeding to trauma processing.

This includes techniques for emotional regulation and distress tolerance, which are essential skills for managing generalized anxiety symptoms. The development of these resources can be an integral part of the EMDR process, providing clients with tools to handle emotional disturbances more effectively.

Addressing Physiological Symptoms: Anxiety disorders are often accompanied by physical symptoms such as heart palpitations, sweating, or dizziness. The body scan phase of EMDR can be particularly beneficial in these cases, helping clients to identify and process somatic experiences associated with their anxiety. This phase allows for the integration of positive beliefs and a sense of safety within the body, reducing the physiological response to anxiety triggers.

Reevaluation and Future Templating: Reevaluation is an ongoing process that assesses the client's progress and adjusts the treatment plan as needed. For individuals with anxiety disorders, this may involve revisiting triggers that continue to provoke anxiety and using future templating to prepare the client for handling these situations more effectively. Future templating involves visualizing oneself successfully coping with potential stressors or anxiety-provoking situations, reinforcing a sense of competence and resilience.

By tailoring the EMDR protocol to address the specific needs of clients with anxiety disorders and phobias, therapists can facilitate a more effective and compassionate treatment process. This approach not only helps in reducing the symptoms of anxiety but also empowers clients to reclaim a sense of control over their lives, fostering lasting change and healing.

8.2: INTEGRATING EMDR FOR DEPRESSION AND ADDICTIONS

Eye Movement Desensitization and Reprocessing (EMDR) therapy has emerged as a powerful tool in the treatment of depression and addictions, complementing traditional therapeutic approaches with its unique methodology. The integration of EMDR into existing treatment plans for mood and addiction disorders can enhance therapeutic outcomes by addressing the underlying trauma that often fuels these conditions. This section delves into the mechanisms through which EMDR augments other therapeutic strategies, providing clinicians with actionable insights for holistic patient care.

EMDR's Role in Treating Depression: Depression is frequently intertwined with past traumatic experiences that shape negative beliefs and self-perceptions. EMDR therapy targets these foundational memories, aiming to reprocess them into less distressing recollections and thereby alleviate depressive symptoms. By incorporating EMDR, therapists can offer a dual approach: while traditional therapies like Cognitive Behavioral Therapy (CBT) tackle the cognitive and behavioral aspects of depression, EMDR focuses on the emotional and traumatic roots, offering a comprehensive treatment strategy.

Enhancing Addiction Treatment: Addictions often serve as maladaptive coping mechanisms for underlying trauma. EMDR therapy aids in the reprocessing of these traumatic memories, reducing the emotional pain that drives the addictive behavior. This process not only addresses the symptomatic layer of addiction but also fosters long-term recovery by resolving the core issues. Integrating EMDR into addiction treatment plans can significantly improve outcomes by providing clients with the tools to manage triggers and cravings more effectively.

Complementing Pharmacotherapy: For many clients, pharmacotherapy is a critical component of managing depression and addictions. EMDR therapy complements this approach by addressing the psychological and emotional dimensions that medication alone cannot reach. This holistic approach ensures that clients receive both the neurochemical support they need and the opportunity to work through the traumas that contribute to their condition.

Collaborative Care Model: Successful integration of EMDR into treatment for depression and addictions requires a collaborative care model. Clinicians should work closely with other healthcare professionals to ensure that EMDR therapy is seamlessly woven into the client's overall treatment plan. This might involve coordinating with psychiatrists, addiction specialists, and other therapists to synchronize treatments and maximize the therapeutic impact.

Tailoring EMDR to Individual Needs: It is crucial to tailor EMDR interventions to suit the specific needs of clients with depression and addictions. This includes careful selection of target memories, pacing the therapy to match the client's readiness, and adjusting the intensity of the bilateral stimulation. Personalizing the EMDR approach ensures that it complements other treatments the client is receiving, enhancing the synergy between different therapeutic modalities.

Monitoring and Adjusting Treatment: Integration of EMDR into broader treatment plans requires ongoing assessment and adjustment. Therapists should closely monitor the client's response to EMDR, particularly how it affects their engagement with other treatments. Regular check-ins and adjustments ensure that the combined therapeutic approaches are optimally supporting the client's recovery journey.

In conclusion, EMDR therapy offers valuable benefits when integrated into treatment plans for depression and addictions, addressing the deep-seated traumas that underlie these conditions. By complementing traditional therapeutic approaches, EMDR can enhance the efficacy of treatment, offering clients a path to more profound and lasting healing. Therapists are encouraged to consider EMDR as a component of a holistic treatment strategy, tailored to meet the unique needs of each client and supported by a collaborative care approach.

8.3: MANAGING CLIENTS WITH SOMATIC SYMPTOMS

In addressing the physical manifestations of trauma through EMDR, therapists encounter a complex interplay between the mind and body. Trauma, particularly when unresolved, often resides not just in the psychological realm but manifests physically in clients. These somatic symptoms can range from chronic pain to gastrointestinal issues, without a clear medical origin. The challenge for therapists is to recognize these symptoms as potential indicators of trauma and to integrate EMDR strategies that can address both psychological and physical distress.

Identifying Somatic Symptoms: The first step is a thorough assessment to differentiate between symptoms that are medically explained and those that might be trauma-related. Common somatic complaints include unexplained chronic pain, headaches, fatigue, and gastrointestinal problems. These symptoms often persist even after medical interventions, suggesting a trauma component.

Integrating the Body Scan Technique: The Body Scan phase of EMDR is crucial for clients with somatic symptoms. This phase allows clients to bring awareness to bodily sensations and to identify areas where trauma might be stored. Therapists guide clients through a process of noticing and describing these sensations without judgment, which can reveal insights into their trauma.

Tailoring Bilateral Stimulation: For clients presenting somatic symptoms, the application of bilateral stimulation requires careful consideration. Adjustments might be needed in the intensity and type of stimulation to ensure it does not exacerbate their physical discomfort. Sometimes, slower and more gentle bilateral stimulation can be more effective in these cases.

Incorporating Somatic Experiencing Techniques: Combining EMDR with somatic experiencing techniques can enhance the therapeutic process for clients with somatic symptoms. Techniques such as grounding and resourcing help clients develop a sense of safety and presence in their bodies, which is often compromised in trauma.

Addressing Negative Cognitions Linked to Somatic Symptoms: Clients may develop negative beliefs about their bodies and their health due to their somatic symptoms. Part of the EMDR process involves identifying and reprocessing these negative cognitions, replacing them with positive, empowering beliefs about the body's ability to heal and regain equilibrium.

Collaboration with Medical Professionals: When treating clients with somatic symptoms, a multidisciplinary approach can be beneficial. Collaboration with medical professionals ensures that clients receive comprehensive care, addressing both the psychological and physiological aspects of their symptoms.

Monitoring and Adjusting the Treatment Plan: Clients with somatic symptoms may require adjustments in their EMDR treatment plan. Frequent check-ins about their physical and emotional responses to therapy can guide necessary modifications in the approach, ensuring that the therapy remains both effective and tolerable.

Fostering Mind-Body Integration: The ultimate goal in treating somatic symptoms with EMDR is to foster integration between mind and body. Helping clients to understand the connection between their trauma and physical symptoms is empowering, paving the way for a more holistic healing process.

Therapists are encouraged to approach clients with somatic symptoms with empathy, patience, and creativity. By carefully adapting EMDR techniques and incorporating somatic practices, therapists can offer a path toward healing that acknowledges the profound interconnectedness of mind and body in trauma recovery.

Part 4:
Real-World Clinical Applications

Chapter 9: Case Studies and Practical Examples

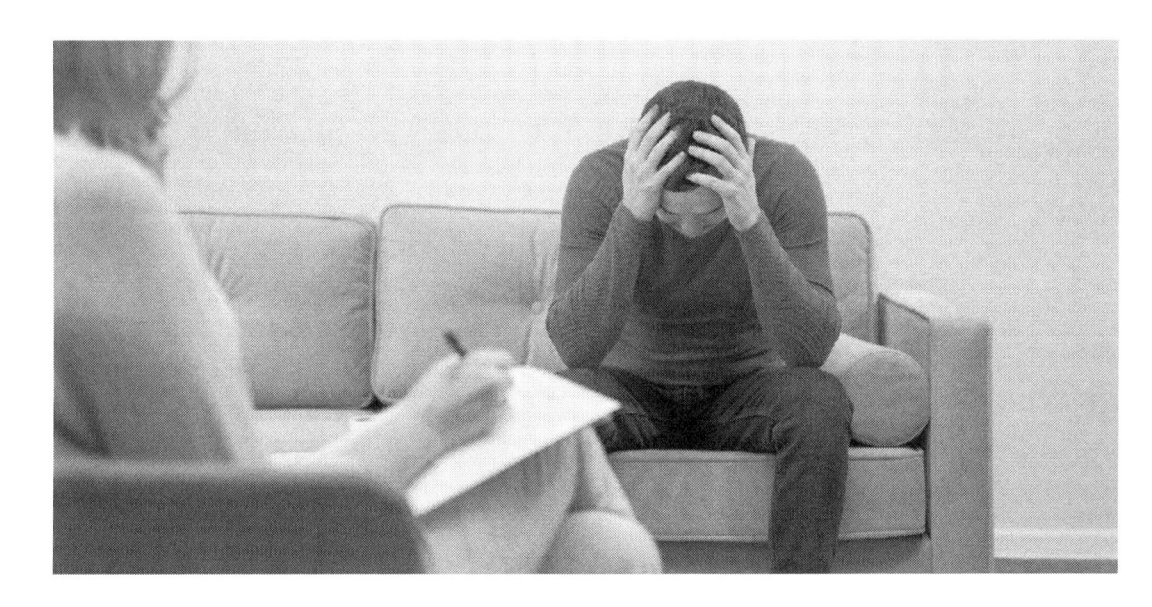

9.1: SINGLE-EVENT TRAUMA TREATMENT IN ADULTS

In treating single-event trauma in an adult client, the therapeutic journey begins with the careful selection of the traumatic memory that will be the focus of the Eye Movement Desensitization and Reprocessing (EMDR) session. This process involves a detailed discussion with the client to identify the event that is most distressing to them. The therapist uses the Subjective Units of Disturbance Scale (SUDS) to gauge the intensity of the emotional disturbance associated with the memory, ensuring that the chosen memory is both relevant and impactful.

Preparation is crucial in setting the stage for a successful EMDR session. The therapist spends time building a strong therapeutic alliance, ensuring the client feels safe and understood. This phase includes educating the client about the EMDR process, what to expect, and how it can help them. Techniques such as deep breathing, visualization, or mindfulness may be introduced to help the client establish a sense of calm and safety, a critical foundation before proceeding to trauma processing.

Assessment involves identifying the negative cognition associated with the traumatic memory, such as "I am powerless" or "I am in danger," and contrasting it with a positive cognition that the client would like to believe instead, like "I am in control" or "I am safe now." The therapist and client collaborate to evaluate the validity of the positive belief on a scale, setting a benchmark for the therapy's progress.

During the **Desensitization** phase, the therapist guides the client through sets of bilateral stimulation, often in the form of side-to-side eye movements, taps, or tones. This stimulation is interspersed with brief pauses to check in on the client's experience. The client is instructed to simply notice whatever spontaneously happens in their mind without attempting to control or analyze the thoughts, images, emotions, or physical sensations that arise. The goal here is to reduce the emotional charge of the memory, as measured by a decrease in SUDS scores.

Installation is the next step, where the focus shifts to strengthening the positive cognition identified earlier. Bilateral stimulation continues, supporting the client in integrating this positive belief into their memory network, effectively replacing the negative cognition. The therapist monitors the client's SUDS scores, ensuring that the emotional disturbance continues to decrease as the positive belief becomes more convincing.

A **Body Scan** is conducted to identify any residual physical tension or discomfort that may be connected to the traumatic memory. The client is asked to mentally scan their body from head to toe, noting any physical sensations. If distress is detected, additional sets of bilateral stimulation are applied until the discomfort is alleviated, further aiding in the resolution of the trauma.

Closure ensures that the client leaves the session feeling better than when they arrived. Regardless of where the client is in the processing of their trauma, the therapist employs techniques to bring them back to a state of equilibrium. This may include revisiting the calming exercises introduced during the preparation phase or discussing a plan for self-care following the session.

Reevaluation occurs at the beginning of the next session, where the therapist assesses the client's current state and the effects of the previous session. This includes revisiting the targeted memory to measure any changes in the SUDS score and the believability of the positive cognition. Based on this assessment, the therapist decides whether further reprocessing of the same memory is needed or if it is time to move on to another target.

This detailed, step-by-step approach to treating single-event trauma with EMDR emphasizes the importance of a structured, phased process that prioritizes the client's safety and emotional stability. By carefully navigating each stage, therapists can help clients reprocess traumatic memories in a way that promotes healing and fosters resilience, ultimately guiding them toward a sense of closure and peace.

9.2: COMPLEX PTSD WITH DISSOCIATION

In treating complex PTSD with dissociation, therapists face the challenge of navigating fragmented memories and the client's fluctuating sense of presence. The advanced Eye Movement Desensitization and Reprocessing (EMDR) strategies tailored for such cases prioritize safety, stabilization, and the gradual integration of dissociated parts of the self. The approach is methodical, requiring the therapist to be highly attuned to the client's needs and responses throughout the therapy.

Grounding Techniques for Stabilization: Before initiating EMDR, it's crucial to establish grounding techniques that the client can reliably use to maintain or return to a sense of present-moment safety. These practices might include focused breathing, sensory engagement exercises, or the use of comforting imagery. Grounding serves as a vital tool for clients to manage dissociative episodes, ensuring they remain anchored during sessions.

Phased Reprocessing Techniques: Given the complex nature of dissociative symptoms, EMDR therapy is often delivered in a phased approach. This begins with the preparation phase, where the therapist and client establish trust and a shared understanding of the treatment goals. Following this, the assessment phase is approached with care, identifying target memories while being mindful of the client's dissociative tendencies. The therapist must be adept at recognizing when a client is becoming overwhelmed or dissociated and be ready to employ grounding techniques as needed.

Fragmented Memories: Clients with complex PTSD may present with memories that are not fully accessible or are experienced as disconnected from their emotional context. The therapist works with the client to gently access these fragmented memories, using EMDR's bilateral stimulation to facilitate processing. This process can help to reconstruct a more cohesive narrative of past events, reducing the distress associated with fragmented recollections.

Integration and Reconnection: A key goal in treating dissociation with EMDR is the integration of dissociated parts and the reconnection of the client with their memories, emotions, and bodily sensations in a safe and controlled manner. This often involves the use of imaginative interweaves, where the therapist introduces concepts or scenarios that encourage the client to integrate experiences or perspectives that were previously dissociated.

Adapting Bilateral Stimulation: In cases of complex PTSD with dissociation, the standard protocol for bilateral stimulation may need to be adapted. This could involve adjusting the speed or intensity of the eye movements or employing alternative forms of bilateral stimulation, such as auditory tones or tactile taps, depending on the client's comfort and response. The therapist's flexibility and creativity in applying these techniques are paramount to facilitating the client's engagement with the process.

Safety and Tolerance Adjustments: Throughout the therapy, the therapist must continuously monitor the client's sense of safety and tolerance for distress. This may necessitate frequent pauses during sessions, the use of shorter bursts of bilateral stimulation, and the incorporation of more extensive grounding and stabilization exercises. The pacing of therapy is deliberately slow and gentle, allowing the client to process traumatic material without becoming overwhelmed.

Collaborative Decision Making: The therapist and client engage in a collaborative process, with the client's feedback guiding the course of treatment. This partnership empowers the client, fostering a sense of agency and control over their healing process. The therapist encourages the client to communicate their needs and boundaries, adjusting the therapy approach in response to the client's experiences and reactions.

Advanced EMDR strategies for treating complex PTSD with dissociation are characterized by their emphasis on safety, stabilization, and a phased approach to processing trauma. Through careful adaptation of techniques and a strong therapeutic alliance, therapists can support clients in navigating the challenges of dissociation, facilitating healing and integration.

9.3: EMDR for First Responders with Chronic PTSD

First responders with chronic PTSD present unique therapeutic challenges due to the nature of their work, which often involves repeated exposure to traumatic events. Tailoring EMDR therapy to meet their specific needs requires a nuanced understanding of these challenges and the implementation of specialized strategies to manage hyperarousal, process occupational trauma, and facilitate long-term emotional regulation. The following strategies are designed to support therapists in this endeavor:

1. Initial Assessment and Stabilization: Begin with a comprehensive assessment to understand the full scope of the first responder's trauma exposure and symptoms. Given the high levels of hyperarousal common among this population, it's crucial to prioritize stabilization techniques early in treatment. Techniques such as diaphragmatic breathing, progressive muscle relaxation, and guided imagery can be effective in reducing immediate symptoms of hyperarousal and preparing the individual for trauma processing.

2. Customizing the Preparation Phase: For first responders, the standard EMDR preparation phase may need to be extended or modified to address the complexities of their trauma and to build a robust repertoire of coping mechanisms. Incorporate psychoeducation about the physiological and psychological impacts of chronic trauma exposure, emphasizing the normalcy of their responses to abnormal events. This can help in reducing self-stigma and promoting a sense of common humanity with others who have endured similar experiences.

3. Selecting and Prioritizing Trauma Targets: When working with first responders, it's important to collaboratively identify and prioritize trauma targets. This process may reveal a pattern of traumatic incidents that are most distressing or a cluster of related traumatic memories. Given the cumulative nature of their trauma exposure, consider starting with more recent incidents before working backward to earlier traumas, unless a specific earlier event is identified as foundational to their PTSD symptoms.

4. Managing Hyperarousal During Reprocessing: Hyperarousal can be a significant barrier to effective reprocessing in first responders. Utilize techniques such as the "float-back" technique to help the individual connect to a specific memory without becoming overwhelmed. Adjust the pace of bilateral stimulation to the individual's tolerance, and be prepared to pause and employ grounding techniques if hyperarousal becomes too intense.

5. Incorporating Occupational Context into Reprocessing: It's essential to acknowledge and integrate the occupational context of the first responder's trauma. This includes recognizing the role of duty and responsibility, the impact of organizational culture, and the possible presence of moral injury. Use cognitive interweaves that validate the individual's experiences and dilemmas faced in the line of duty, and help them reframe self-critical beliefs related to their trauma.

6. Enhancing Emotional Regulation: Long-term emotional regulation is a critical goal for first responders with chronic PTSD. Throughout the EMDR process, emphasize the development of skills for managing emotional responses to triggers. This can include the integration of mindfulness practices, emotion regulation strategies from Dialectical Behavior Therapy (DBT), and techniques for modulating physiological arousal.

7. Addressing Secondary Traumatization: Recognize and address signs of secondary traumatization, which can arise from the cumulative impact of exposure to the suffering of others. This aspect of their trauma may require specific attention during the reprocessing phases of EMDR, with a focus on desensitizing distressing images and beliefs about helplessness or failure to save others.

8. Supporting Occupational Identity and Resilience: Work with the first responder to explore and reinforce a sense of positive occupational identity and resilience. This includes acknowledging the strengths and coping strategies that have allowed them to perform their roles effectively, as well as fostering a sense of accomplishment and pride in their work.

9. Planning for Future Stressors: Finally, prepare the first responder for future stressors and potential triggers related to their work. Develop a comprehensive plan that includes early recognition of symptoms, strategies for immediate coping and self-regulation, and a clear protocol for seeking additional support if needed.

By carefully adapting EMDR therapy to the specific needs of first responders with chronic PTSD, therapists can provide targeted support that addresses the complexities of occupational trauma, manages symptoms of hyperarousal, and promotes long-term emotional regulation and resilience. This tailored approach not only facilitates the processing of traumatic memories but also supports first responders in continuing their vital work with a renewed sense of strength and well-being.

Part 5: The EMDR Therapist's Toolkit

Chapter 10: Scripts for EMDR Sessions

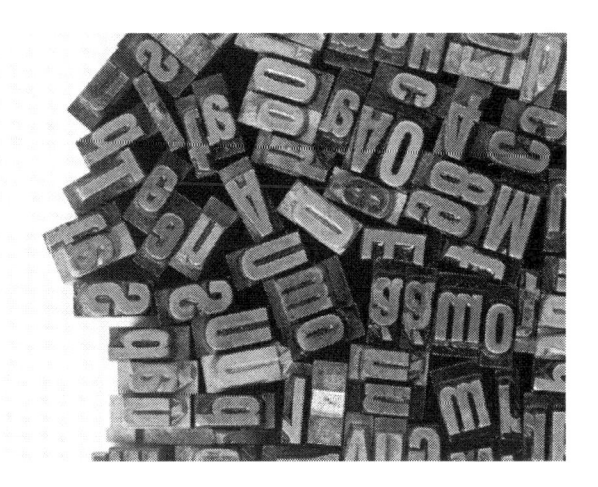

10.1: Safe/Calm Place Script

In this script, we guide the client to establish a **safe/calm place**, which is a foundational exercise in emotional stabilization. This mental space serves as a refuge, where the client can retreat to feel secure and at peace, especially when navigating through the challenges of processing traumatic memories. The creation and utilization of this safe place are critical in preparing clients for the deeper work of EMDR therapy.

Step 1: Setting the Scene: Begin by inviting the client to find a comfortable position, encouraging them to close their eyes if they feel comfortable doing so. Guide them to take a few deep breaths, focusing on the sensation of air filling their lungs and the relaxation that follows each exhale. This initial step is crucial for grounding and centering the client in the present moment.

Step 2: Visualization: Next, instruct the client to envision a place where they feel completely safe and calm. This place can be real or imagined, indoors or outdoors. The key is that it feels secure, peaceful, and comforting to them. Encourage them to notice the details of this place—the colors, sounds, textures, and any scents that might be present. The more vivid the description, the more real the place will feel.

Step 3: Engaging the Senses: Encourage the client to engage all their senses as they continue to explore their safe place. What do they hear? Is there a gentle breeze or the sound of waves crashing? What do they see? Bright sunlight filtering through leaves or the soft glow of lamps? What do they feel? The warmth of the sun or the coolness of shade? What do they smell? Freshly cut grass or salty sea air? Engaging the senses deepens the experience and reinforces the feeling of safety.

Step 4: Emotional Anchoring: Once the client has fully immersed themselves in their safe place, guide them to connect with the feelings of safety, peace, and calm that this place provides. Ask them to notice where in their body they feel these sensations the most. Encourage them to amplify these feelings, imagining them spreading throughout their body, anchoring them in this sense of safety and calm.

Step 5: Creating a Mental Snapshot: Instruct the client to take a mental snapshot of their safe place, capturing all the details and the feelings associated with it. This snapshot will serve as a quick-access point that they can return to whenever they need a moment of peace or feel overwhelmed during therapy or in daily life.

Step 6: Returning to the Present: Finally, guide the client to slowly bring their awareness back to the present room, encouraging them to bring the feelings of safety and calm with them. Remind them that their safe place is always accessible to them whenever they need it, simply by closing their eyes and revisiting their mental snapshot.

This script is a powerful tool in the EMDR therapist's toolkit, providing clients with a personal refuge that supports emotional regulation and readiness for trauma processing. It is an essential component of preparation for EMDR therapy, ensuring that clients have a means of self-soothing and stabilization as they work through their traumatic memories.

10.2 GROUNDING TECHNIQUES FOR DISSOCIATIVE CLIENTS

Objective: To provide therapists with effective grounding techniques specifically designed for clients experiencing dissociation, aiming to enhance their present-moment awareness and reduce the intensity of dissociative episodes during EMDR therapy sessions.

Step-by-step instructions:

1. **Sensory Engagement:**

    - Encourage the client to engage all five senses one by one. Ask them to identify one thing they can see, one sound they can hear, one object they can touch, one scent they can smell, and if appropriate, one taste. This helps in anchoring them to the present moment.

2. **Breathing Techniques:**

    - Instruct the client to focus on their breath, guiding them to inhale deeply through the nose for a count of four, hold for a count of four, and exhale slowly through the mouth for a count of six. This pattern helps regulate the nervous system and decreases dissociative symptoms.

3. **Temperature Awareness:**

    - Offer the client a cold water bottle to hold or a warm blanket to wrap around themselves. The sensation of cold or warmth can serve as a physical anchor, bringing their awareness back to the present and away from dissociative thoughts.

4. **Focused Attention:**

   - Ask the client to pick an object in the room and describe it in detail, including its color, shape, texture, and any other observable features. This exercise helps shift focus from internal distress to external reality.

5. **Movement and Stretching:**

   - Guide the client through simple, gentle stretching exercises or encourage them to stand up and move around the space if appropriate. Physical movement can help dissipate stored energy and reduce feelings of being 'stuck' in a dissociative state.

6. **Sound Orientation:**

   - Use a soft bell or chime to create a gentle sound. Ask the client to listen closely to the sound and raise their hand when they can no longer hear it. This practice helps enhance auditory focus and present-moment awareness.

7. **Guided Imagery for Grounding:**

   - Lead the client through a guided imagery exercise where they imagine roots growing from the soles of their feet deep into the earth, grounding them firmly to the present. This visualization promotes a sense of stability and connectedness.

8. **Use of Affirmations:**

   - Encourage the client to repeat affirmations that foster a sense of safety and presence, such as "I am here," "I am safe," or "I am in control." Affirmations can be personalized to resonate more deeply with the client's experiences.

9. **Aromatherapy:**

   - If available and with the client's consent, introduce calming scents using essential oils or scented lotion. Ask the client to focus on the scent, which can serve as a pleasant and grounding sensory input.

10. **Visual Focus Exercise:**

- Invite the client to focus on a specific point in the room, such as a spot on the wall or a particular object. Instruct them to maintain their gaze on this point while taking deep, slow breaths, helping to stabilize their attention and reduce dissociation.

Each technique can be individually tailored to the client's preferences and responses, ensuring the most effective grounding experience during EMDR sessions.

10.3: INSTALLATION AND BODY SCAN SCRIPTS

In the process of EMDR therapy, the installation phase is crucial for reinforcing positive beliefs that counterbalance the client's negative cognitions. This phase is closely followed by the body scan, which helps identify and resolve any residual somatic distress linked to traumatic memories. Here, we provide detailed scripts for both installation and body scan phases, designed to facilitate healing and integration for clients.

Installation Phase Script

1. Begin by reminding the client of the positive cognition (PC) they have chosen to replace their negative belief. Ensure that the PC feels true and powerful to them, even if only slightly at this moment.

2. Ask the client to bring up the target memory that has been the focus of the session. Encourage them to hold this memory in mind alongside the positive belief.

3. Initiate bilateral stimulation, using the method that has been most effective for the client, whether it be eye movements, taps, or tones.

4. After each set of bilateral stimulation, pause to ask the client to let you know what they noticed, without aiming to guide their thoughts or feelings in any specific direction.

5. Continue with the bilateral stimulation, interspersing with check-ins, until the client reports that the positive cognition feels fully true when thinking about the target memory. Use the Validity of Cognition (VOC) scale to measure how true the positive belief feels, aiming for a score as close to 7 as possible.

6. Throughout this phase, maintain a supportive and validating presence, acknowledging the client's progress and reinforcing the strength of the positive cognition.

Body Scan Script

1. Once the installation of the positive cognition is complete, transition to the body scan by asking the client to close their eyes, if they're comfortable doing so, and take a few deep breaths to center themselves.

2. Instruct the client to mentally scan their body from head to toe, noticing any areas of tension, discomfort, or unusual sensations. Emphasize that there's no right or wrong thing to notice; the goal is simply to become aware of bodily sensations.

3. If the client identifies any areas of distress, use a focused set of bilateral stimulation to target these sensations. Ask the client to concentrate on the physical discomfort while engaging in the bilateral stimulation.

4. After each set of bilateral stimulation, inquire about any changes in the sensation. It may increase, decrease, move, or change in quality — any of these responses is normal.

5. Continue the process until the client reports no distressing bodily sensations or until the sensations have significantly reduced in intensity.

6. Conclude the body scan by inviting the client to take a few more deep breaths and, when ready, to open their eyes, bringing their awareness back to the present moment and the safety of the therapeutic environment.

These scripts are designed to be flexible and adaptable to each client's unique needs and responses. The goal of the installation phase is to solidify the client's connection to positive beliefs, thereby enhancing their resilience against traumatic memories. The body scan, meanwhile, aims to release any residual physical tension or discomfort, ensuring a comprehensive approach to trauma treatment. Through these carefully structured scripts, therapists can guide their clients towards a deeper healing process, addressing both cognitive and somatic components of trauma.

10.4: INCORPORATING TECHNOLOGY INTO EMDR SESSIONS

In the realm of EMDR therapy, the integration of technology and digital tools has emerged as a transformative approach, enhancing the therapeutic experience and outcomes for clients. This section delves into practical instructions for embedding these innovations into session scripts, ensuring therapists can leverage technology to its fullest potential.

Digital Tools for Bilateral Stimulation: The core of EMDR therapy involves bilateral stimulation, traditionally conducted through eye movements, auditory tones, or tactile taps. Modern advancements have introduced digital applications capable of delivering this stimulation with precision and flexibility. Therapists can utilize apps that control the speed, intensity, and pattern of stimulation, allowing for a customized experience tailored to each client's needs. Incorporating these apps into sessions can be as simple as connecting a device to speakers for auditory stimulation or a screen for visual cues, ensuring the client is comfortable and the settings are adjusted to their preference.

Virtual Reality (VR) for Immersive Environments: VR technology offers an unparalleled opportunity to create immersive environments that can facilitate the EMDR process. By using VR headsets, therapists can place clients in settings that promote relaxation and safety, such as a peaceful beach or serene forest. These environments can be particularly beneficial during the Preparation phase, helping clients establish a calm place mentally. Furthermore, VR can be employed to simulate scenarios related to the target memory in a controlled manner, enhancing the Assessment and Desensitization phases.

Online Platforms for Remote EMDR Sessions: The rise of teletherapy has necessitated the adaptation of EMDR to online formats. Platforms specifically designed for remote EMDR sessions enable therapists to conduct therapy with clients who are not physically present in the office. These platforms often come equipped with built-in tools for bilateral stimulation and secure communication channels, ensuring the therapy's effectiveness is maintained.

Therapists should familiarize themselves with these platforms, ensuring they can navigate the tools efficiently and provide clear instructions to clients for a seamless experience.

Apps for Client Self-Regulation and Homework: Engaging clients in their healing process outside of sessions is crucial for the success of EMDR therapy. Numerous apps offer guided exercises for relaxation, mindfulness, and emotional regulation, which clients can use as homework. Therapists should recommend specific apps that align with the therapeutic goals, providing clients with resources to practice skills like grounding and mindfulness. These tools not only empower clients but also reinforce the progress made during sessions.

Data Tracking and Progress Monitoring Tools: Keeping track of a client's progress is essential for adjusting treatment plans and measuring outcomes. Digital tools and software designed for therapists can facilitate this process by allowing the collection of data on clients' symptomatology, session feedback, and homework completion. Therapists can integrate these tools into their practice, ensuring that they have access to comprehensive data that informs their therapeutic decisions. Regularly reviewing this data with clients can also enhance their engagement and motivation in the therapy process.

Incorporating technology into EMDR sessions represents a forward-thinking approach that aligns with contemporary clinical practices. By embracing these tools, therapists can enhance the efficacy of EMDR, offering clients innovative and effective means of processing trauma. It is crucial, however, to ensure that any technology used is in service of the therapeutic goals and is implemented in a way that respects the client's comfort and readiness. As the field of EMDR continues to evolve, staying informed about technological advancements and integrating them thoughtfully into therapy will remain a key component of effective trauma treatment.

10.5: GUIDED MINDFULNESS SCRIPTS FOR TRAUMA

Mindfulness practices offer a powerful complement to the Eye Movement Desensitization and Reprocessing (EMDR) framework, especially for clients grappling with trauma and dissociation. These practices aim to anchor individuals in the present moment, fostering a sense of safety and bodily awareness that can be particularly beneficial for those who have experienced trauma. The following script is designed to be integrated into EMDR sessions, providing clients with tools to manage trauma responses and enhance their connection to their physical selves.

Engaging the Breath as an Anchor

Begin by inviting your client to find a comfortable seated or lying position, encouraging them to adjust their posture until they feel at ease. Guide them to place one hand on their abdomen and the other on their chest, feeling the rise and fall with each breath. This tactile connection serves as a direct link to the present moment, grounding the client in their bodily sensations.

Focusing on the Senses

Direct the client's attention to their immediate environment, asking them to identify and name three things they can see, three sounds they can hear, and three textures they can feel. This exercise draws their awareness outward, away from internal distress and towards the external world, reinforcing their sense of safety and control.

Body Scan for Presence

Encourage the client to mentally scan their body from head to toe, noting any areas of tension, discomfort, or numbness. This practice not only promotes present-moment awareness but also allows the client to reconnect with their body in a gentle, non-judgmental way. Remind them that they have the power to bring kindness and curiosity to their experience, fostering a healing relationship with their physical self.

Mindful Movement to Release Trauma

Introduce simple, mindful movements, such as stretching the arms overhead or gently twisting the torso, guiding the client to move with intention and awareness. These movements can help release stored tension and trauma in the body, making them particularly useful for clients who experience dissociation. Emphasize the importance of moving within the comfort zone and listening to the body's signals.

Visualization for Self-Compassion

Guide your client through a visualization exercise where they imagine a warm, soothing light enveloping them, representing compassion and safety. Encourage them to visualize this light healing any wounds, both physical and emotional, and to see themselves with kindness and understanding. This practice can help shift self-perception from one of victimhood to one of resilience and self-compassion.

Breathing Space for Emotional Regulation

Teach the client the "Three-Minute Breathing Space" exercise, which involves spending one minute focusing on the breath, one minute on bodily sensations, and one minute on thoughts and emotions. This technique offers a quick and effective way for clients to center themselves during moments of distress, providing a sense of control over their emotional responses.

Gratitude Reflection

Conclude the mindfulness practice by inviting the client to reflect on aspects of their life they are grateful for. This shift in focus towards gratitude can help counterbalance the negative bias often found in trauma survivors, promoting positive emotions and a broader perspective on life.

Incorporating these mindfulness scripts into EMDR therapy sessions can significantly enhance the therapeutic process for clients dealing with trauma and dissociation. By fostering a stronger connection to the present moment and their bodies, clients can develop resilience against trauma responses, laying the foundation for deeper healing.

Chapter 11: Advanced Target Selection for EMDR

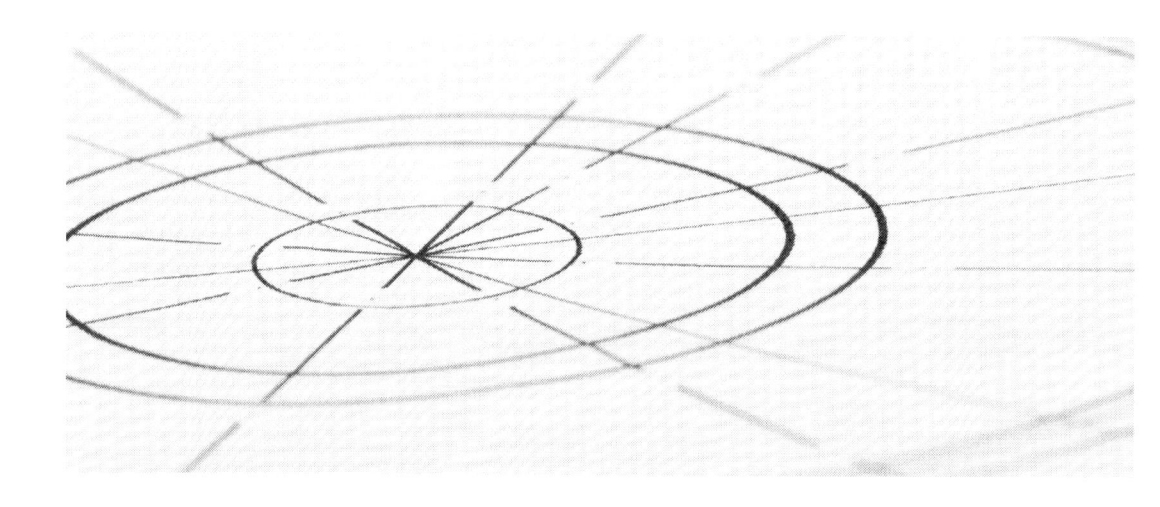

11.1: Understanding Target Selection in EMDR

The principles of target selection in EMDR therapy are foundational to its effectiveness in treating trauma. This process involves a meticulous evaluation of the client's experiences to identify specific memories that serve as the basis for trauma-related symptoms. The goal is to prioritize these memories for therapeutic attention, ensuring a structured approach to healing. The Adaptive Information Processing (AIP) model posits that psychological stress is the result of unprocessed memories. Therefore, the selection of targets is critical in facilitating the processing of these memories, leading to symptom relief and improved mental health.

Past Trauma: Identifying past traumatic events is the first step in target selection. These are incidents that continue to exert a negative influence on the client's emotional well-being and daily functioning. It is essential to gather a comprehensive history of these events, understanding their context, the emotions involved, and the impact on the individual's life. This historical overview aids in constructing a timeline of trauma, which is invaluable in prioritizing which memories to target first. Often, the focus begins with early traumas, under the premise that processing these foundational experiences can significantly reduce the intensity of later trauma symptoms.

Present Triggers: Present triggers are current situations, environments, or stimuli that provoke a distressing response due to their association with past trauma. Identifying these triggers is crucial as they offer insight into how unprocessed memories are influencing the client's current emotional state and behavior. By understanding these triggers, therapists can more effectively tailor EMDR interventions to address the specific contexts that are problematic for the client. This approach not only aids in desensitizing the client to these triggers but also in reprocessing the underlying memories that fuel their power.

Future Concerns: Future concerns involve anticipated situations that evoke fear or anxiety in the client, often as a projection of past trauma onto future possibilities. These concerns can significantly impair the client's ability to function and engage with life positively. By identifying these anxieties, therapists can use EMDR to help clients develop more adaptive coping mechanisms and beliefs about their future. This aspect of target selection is oriented towards enhancing the client's resilience and capacity to envision a future where they are not defined or limited by their trauma.

In selecting targets for EMDR therapy, it is important to adopt a phased approach, starting with past traumas, moving through present triggers, and addressing future concerns. This structured progression ensures a comprehensive treatment plan that facilitates healing across the client's temporal experience of trauma. Additionally, therapists should remain flexible, responsive to the client's evolving needs as therapy progresses. The ultimate aim is to empower clients, enabling them to process their traumatic memories and reduce their symptomatic distress, thereby improving their quality of life.

11.2: CLUSTERED TARGET APPROACH FOR COMPLEX TRAUMA

The Clustered Target Approach for complex trauma involves organizing interconnected traumatic memories into clusters, allowing for a more structured and effective EMDR treatment process. This approach acknowledges that individuals with complex trauma often have multiple traumatic memories that are densely interconnected, influencing their current psychological state. By identifying and grouping these memories, therapists can address the trauma more holistically, facilitating deeper healing.

Identifying Memory Clusters: The first step is to work with the client to map out the traumatic memories, identifying patterns or themes that emerge. These could be based on the nature of the trauma, the emotional response they elicit, or the life period in which they occurred. This process not only aids in organizing the treatment plan but also helps the client and therapist understand the breadth and depth of the trauma.

Prioritizing Clusters for Treatment: Once clusters have been identified, the next step is to prioritize them for treatment. This decision should be based on several factors, including the client's current symptoms, the intensity of the emotional distress associated with each cluster, and the client's treatment goals. Starting with clusters that are foundational to the client's trauma narrative can often create significant shifts in their psychological well-being, making subsequent clusters easier to address.

Sequential Reprocessing: After prioritization, the therapist and client engage in the sequential reprocessing of each cluster. This involves working through the memories within a cluster using EMDR therapy, starting with the earliest or most impactful memories as determined during the prioritization phase. Sequential reprocessing allows for the thorough processing of all aspects of the trauma, reducing the likelihood of retraumatization and ensuring a comprehensive treatment approach.

Integration of Positive Cognitions: As each cluster is reprocessed, it is crucial to integrate positive cognitions that counteract the negative beliefs stemming from the traumatic memories. This step is essential for transforming the client's self-perception and their understanding of the traumatic events, fostering a sense of empowerment and resilience.

Evaluating Progress and Adjusting the Treatment Plan: Throughout the clustered target approach, continuous evaluation of the client's progress is necessary. This involves assessing changes in symptoms, emotional regulation, and the client's overall sense of well-being. Based on these evaluations, adjustments to the treatment plan, such as re-prioritizing clusters or revisiting previously processed memories, may be required to ensure optimal outcomes.

Addressing Residual Effects: Even after the reprocessing of memory clusters, some clients may experience residual effects of the trauma. In these cases, additional EMDR sessions focusing on these lingering symptoms or incorporating other therapeutic interventions may be beneficial. This holistic approach ensures that the treatment addresses all aspects of the client's trauma, facilitating a more complete recovery.

By employing the clustered target approach in EMDR therapy, therapists can provide a structured and comprehensive treatment for individuals with complex trauma. This methodical strategy not only enhances the effectiveness of the therapy but also supports clients in navigating their healing journey with greater clarity and confidence.

11.3: ADDRESSING IMPLICIT AND NON-VERBAL MEMORIES

Implicit and non-verbal memories pose a unique challenge in trauma therapy, particularly when utilizing Eye Movement Desensitization and Reprocessing (EMDR). These memories, often stored without clear imagery or verbal content, can significantly impact a client's emotional and physical well-being. Recognizing and processing these types of memories require specialized approaches that go beyond traditional verbal narrative techniques.

Firstly, it's crucial to understand that implicit memories may manifest through physical sensations, emotions, or behaviors rather than explicit recollections. Clients might experience unexplained anxiety, fear, or somatic symptoms without a clear memory of the original traumatic event. This phenomenon underscores the importance of a therapist's ability to detect subtle cues that indicate the presence of implicit memories.

Techniques for Identifying Implicit Memories

1. **Somatic Tracking**: Encourage clients to become attuned to their bodily sensations. This process involves guiding them to notice and describe any physical sensations, no matter how minor or unrelated they may seem. Somatic tracking can reveal patterns or triggers related to implicit memories.

2. **Emotion Bridging**: Use current emotional reactions as a bridge to access implicit memories. When clients present with strong emotional responses that seem disproportionate to the current situation, explore these emotions to uncover underlying memories.

3. **Behavioral Clues**: Observe clients' behaviors and reactions in therapy. Automatic responses, such as flinching at sudden movements or experiencing distress with specific sounds, can provide clues to implicit memories.

Processing Techniques for Implicit Memories

Once implicit memories are identified, processing them through EMDR can be challenging due to their non-verbal nature. The following strategies can facilitate the processing of these memories:

- **Bilateral Stimulation without Direct Recall**: Engage clients in bilateral stimulation while they focus on the physical sensation or emotion linked to the implicit memory. This approach allows for processing without the need for explicit recall of the traumatic event.

- **Resource Installation**: Strengthen clients' internal resources before attempting to process implicit memories. Techniques such as the safe/calm place exercise can enhance clients' ability to tolerate distressing emotions or sensations that arise during processing.

- **Creative Expression**: Encourage non-verbal forms of expression, such as drawing, music, or movement, to help clients externalize and process implicit memories. These activities can provide a bridge to verbal processing and integration of the memories.

- **Body Scan**: After bilateral stimulation, use the body scan technique to help clients identify and process any residual physical sensations associated with the implicit memory. This step is crucial for ensuring that the processing is comprehensive.

Incorporating these techniques into EMDR therapy requires patience, sensitivity, and flexibility. Therapists must remain attuned to their clients' responses and adjust their approach as needed. The goal is to facilitate the integration of implicit memories into the client's narrative in a way that promotes healing and resolution. By acknowledging and addressing the complexity of implicit and non-verbal memories, therapists can support their clients in achieving a more profound and lasting recovery.

11.4: TARGETING SOMATIC EXPERIENCES IN EMDR

In addressing the complexities of trauma, therapists often encounter clients whose experiences are deeply entrenched not just in their minds but also in their bodies. Somatic experiences, or the physical sensations associated with traumatic memories, can persist long after the event has passed, manifesting as tension, pain, or other discomforts without an apparent physical cause. These sensations are critical cues, signaling areas of unprocessed trauma within the body. To effectively target these somatic experiences in EMDR therapy, a nuanced approach is required, one that respects the intricate connection between body and mind.

The first step in this process involves the identification of somatic experiences. This can be achieved through a detailed client history and a keen observation of the client's nonverbal cues during sessions. Therapists should encourage clients to attune to their bodies, noting any physical sensations that arise when recalling or discussing traumatic events. This practice of somatic awareness can be facilitated through guided exercises that help clients become more mindful of their bodily states.

Once somatic experiences are identified, therapists can employ a variety of strategies to process these physical sensations. One effective approach is the incorporation of bilateral stimulation while the client focuses on the somatic sensation itself, rather than the narrative of the traumatic event. This method allows the client to process the trauma stored in the body without becoming overwhelmed by the emotional and cognitive aspects of the memory.

Another key strategy involves the use of the body scan technique following bilateral stimulation. This technique encourages clients to mentally scan their body from head to toe, noting any areas of tension, discomfort, or other sensations. By bringing awareness to these sensations and using EMDR techniques to process them, clients can begin to release the physical manifestations of trauma.

It is also beneficial to integrate resource installation early in the therapy process to build a foundation of internal safety and stability. Techniques such as the safe/calm place exercise can be particularly useful for clients who struggle with intense somatic responses. Establishing a sense of safety and calm within the body creates a supportive environment for processing traumatic memories.

In some cases, therapists may find it helpful to incorporate adjunctive therapies that focus on somatic experiences, such as somatic experiencing or sensorimotor psychotherapy. These approaches can complement EMDR by providing additional pathways to access and process trauma stored in the body.

Throughout this process, it is vital for therapists to maintain a posture of curiosity, openness, and non-judgment. Encouraging clients to explore the sensations in their bodies without fear or avoidance can lead to significant breakthroughs in therapy. By validating the client's experience and supporting them through the processing of somatic experiences, therapists can help clients achieve a deeper level of healing and integration.

In conclusion, targeting somatic experiences in EMDR requires a thoughtful and multifaceted approach. By recognizing the importance of the body in trauma therapy and employing strategies to address somatic experiences, therapists can facilitate a more comprehensive and holistic healing process for their clients.

Made in United States
Orlando, FL
07 June 2025